Leadership and Nursing

ESSENTIALS OF NURSING MANAGEMENT

Series Editor: Jill Baker

The complexity and changing status of the National Health Service demands that all key professional staff are accountable for both their practice and for the efficient and effective deployment of human and physical resources. The series equips nurses and midwives with the knowledge and skills essential for the application of effective managerial and leadership practice. The series focuses on a range of significant management issues that confront and challenge practising nurses, managers and educationalists working within both hospital and primary care settings.

All books in the series:

Clinical Supervision in Practice: Some Questions, Answers and Guidelines for Professionals in Health and Social Care, 2ed
Edited by Veronica Bishop

Financial Management: Budgeting in Hospitals and Primary Care Trusts 2ed
by Matthew Cripps, Alan Stuttard and Geoffrey Woodhall

Managing Yourself, 2nd edition
by Verena Tschudin and Jane Schober

Leadership and Nursing
by June Girvin

Managing Change, 2ed
by Annabel Broome

Quality Assurance, 2ed
by Diana Sale

Essentials of Nursing Management Series
Series Standing Order
ISBN 1-4039-4597-7
(outside North America only)

You can receive future titles in this series as they are published by placing a standing order. Please contact your bookseller or, in case of difficulty, write to us at the address below with your name and address, the title of the series and the ISBN quoted above.

Customer Services Department, Macmillan Distribution Ltd
Houndmills, Basingstoke, Hampshire RG21 6XS, England

ESSENTIALS OF NURSING MANAGEMENT

Leadership and Nursing

June Girvin

palgrave

Published by
PALGRAVE
Houndmills, Basingstoke, Hampshire RG21 6XS and
175 Fifth Avenue, New York, N. Y. 10010
Companies and representatives throughout the world

PALGRAVE is the new global academic imprint of
St. Martin's Press LLC Scholarly and Reference Division and
Palgrave Publishers Ltd (formerly Macmillan Press Ltd).

ISBN-13: 978-0-333-72375-3
ISBN-10: 0-333-72375-9

This book is printed on paper suitable for recycling and made from fully managed and sustained forest sources.

A catalogue record for this book is available from the British Library.

10   9
07   06

Editing and origination by
Aardvark Editorial, Mendham, Suffolk

Printed in China

For the members of PNF 1993–1996

Contents

Contents

Acknowledgements

There are many people who have been instrumental in the development and formation of this book, those mentioned below having made a particular contribution.

Special thanks go to Mary Monnington, who has proved to be a friend indeed. She also makes me laugh, which has been an especially useful talent over the past 2 years! Thanks also go to Professor Steven West of the University of the West of England who has been generous with his time and his advice, and who eased the pressures on me at just the right moments. I am truly grateful to you both.

Thanks are due to Steph Keeble and Liz Tregoing for reading and commenting on the early drafts – especially to Liz for the hospitality enjoyed in her beautiful Cotswold garden and for the many sensible suggestions that she made for improving the text. I would also like to thank my husband, Adrian, who is always there, whatever happens.

Preface

This book has been written during what can at best be described as a challenging period in my career, but a period in which I have learned much about leadership. Writing it has helped me to make sense of many experiences – not just recent ones, but also ones from throughout my career – and I hope that it will also help the reader to see things a little more clearly. Good leadership is a beacon in a murky world. It can make even the most difficult of circumstances exciting and stimulating to work through. Good leaders should be nurtured, supported and recognised for the major contribution they can make to working lives. Poor leadership not only stunts organisations, but can also leave the people working in those organisations angry, frustrated and bewildered.

Sadly, our tolerance of ineffective leadership seems endless, particularly where it occurs outside our own profession. We have been, and still are, quick to criticise nurse leaders who do not meet our expectations, but it is harder to be openly critical of the hand that feeds us – the manager and the employer. Recognising poor leadership is the first step towards improving it. This book is written to help nurses to understand nursing leadership and the factors that have influenced its development over the years, but I hope that it may also enable the reader to recognise good and not so good leadership, whatever the background of the leader. I hope that it helps readers to choose their role models carefully and develop their own skills effectively.

In an ideal world, I would dearly like to see a clinical qualification become essential for any senior, influential management position. Clinicians are best placed to manage and lead the service; they do, after all, know it best. Far too few nurses aspire to chief executive positions, and even fewer actually reach them. Nursing is not a support service, but it is a hard struggle ensuring that it is not treated like one. So, learn to lead – then get out there and turn the boardroom tables over.

JMG
September 1997

Introduction

Leadership. It has seemed recently that we cannot open a nursing journal without this word leaping out at us. We all seem to want it. Some of us want to provide it. Judging by the debate that goes on in the aforementioned journals, it appears that many people think that nursing needs more of it. But what is this thing called leadership? And what is good or effective nursing leadership?

When we come into contact with good leadership, whether it is our own or someone else's, we are able to recognise it immediately, but ask us to describe it and our terms are nebulous and subjective. Bennis and Nanus (1986) claim that leadership is the most studied and least understood topic in the whole of social science. My own experiences confirm this. A few years ago, I studied leadership and nursing for a Master of Science degree. Once I had explored the general literature on leadership (of which there is a huge amount) and turned to the literature specific to leadership and nursing, I found (certainly in the British literature) – not very much. What did make itself apparent was a yearning in nursing for some kind of 'Holy Grail' called 'leadership'. According to the nursing literature over the past decade or so, we need more leadership, or at least we need better leadership. We do not seem to have enough leaders of the 'right' sort – whatever that may be. I read many opinions and suggestions and, at times, some angry words on how the profession was failing to develop the leaders it needs. However, there was little that described good leadership or explored leadership in any detail. Nursing, with this constant striving for new and better leaders, seems to reflect the problems that have been commonly associated with perceptions of leadership as outlined by Bennis and Nanus: increased complexity of organisations and processes, a lack of commitment in the workforce resulting from shifting

1

social values which foster mobility and multiple career patterns, and a decreasing faith in leaders of all kinds that stems from the public reporting of unethical behaviour. As a professional group, our dissatisfaction with our leaders is a reaction to problems that beset the whole of our working society.

Having said that, there is an increasing amount of literature, much of it from the USA, that concentrates on nursing leadership, but there is still a long way to go. There is a more constructive and structured interest in nursing leadership through work by the King's Fund and the Royal College of Nursing, and some regions of the National Health Service (NHS) Executive have developed leadership programmes. I hope that these initiatives will lead to a recognition of the specific and special skills required by those who hope to lead and also to the facilitation of those skills. My fear is that they may become confused with management skills and training. Only time, and the performance of the leaders coming out of such programmes, will tell.

In most organisations today – including health care organisations – stability and security are highly desirable and highly prized. Organisations do all that they can to protect themselves from risk and reduce any threat of instability (Porter-O'Grady 1992). These organisations tend to choose their managers or leaders because of their ability to reduce risk and maintain stability. Unfortunately, this does not fit well with the requirements for change and innovation that today's health care organisations require in order to meet the needs of patients and clients. This conflict of stability and security versus risk and creativity appears to be the cause of a great deal of tension in management teams all around the NHS, as the few who understand the new ways of 'leading' battle it out with those who want to hold on to the old ways of 'controlling'. Developing leaders who will be able to surge through this and go on to transform our working and caring environments is crucial for the well-being of patients and nurses. In order for this to happen, we must understand what leadership means in reality and what has moulded that reality.

My personal experiences of exploring leadership, especially leadership in nursing, have made me want to share some of the findings with a wider audience. I wanted to encourage a continuing debate on what leadership really means and what the skills, activities and behaviours of a good leader are. Much of what I discovered in the course of this exploration was not new. There were theories that had been around for a very long time in some cases, but I had never taken much interest in them before. My exploration led me into history, politics, sociology and gender studies. This work was fascinating and is helping me to develop a better understanding of why nursing continually cries out for better leaders and better leadership.

By understanding how nursing has been shaped and moulded by history, politics and the struggle for power in organisations, I began to understand why leadership skills were so crucial and what some of those skills needed to be. Exploring the past gives a better understanding of the reactions and attitudes of colleagues to me as a nurse leader. It means I can positively consider appropriate strategies for expressing my own leadership. During the course of my career, I have held a variety of jobs recognised as leadership positions – staff nurse, sister, senior nurse, nurse executive. Some of these posts were within a managerial structure, some outside. With hindsight, there are a number of things that would have helped me in those jobs had I been more aware of them, for example, being taught during training about leadership theory and behaviours, paying more attention to nursing history, a better understanding of the politics of health care reorganisations when they were taking place, and an earlier interest in gender issues.

The purpose of this book is to set out simply some of the things I wish I had known a long time ago. They have helped me enormously as I have discovered them over the years, especially in putting them all together to see how one affected another. If, when you have read this book, you see things in a different light and are able, as a result, to recognise and plan different leadership strategies, it will have been worthwhile. I hope that this book will be used as a basis for discussion and to identify behaviours in our environment. Most of the chapters contain discussion points, which are intended to stimulate thinking about the concept of leadership and the issues that surround it. They will be useful to you as starting points for group discussions or seminar work. In addition, any readers who wish to contact me with personal views and thoughts can do so via the publishers. I hope that the debate continues for a long time to come and that we can continuously improve how we prepare ourselves for leading in our profession and in our health services.

References

Bennis W and Nanus B (1986) *Leaders: The Strategies for Taking Charge.* Harper & Row. London.

Porter-O'Grady T (1992) Transformational leadership in an age of chaos. *Nursing Administration Quarterly.* **17**(1): 17–24.

Chapter 1 The Development of Theories of Leadership

The first three chapters of this book aim to give a sense of how leadership, and the study of it, has evolved over the years – from the earliest writings to the recent past, paying particular attention to the period from the 1940s when studies became more focused and systematic. The remaining chapters look at more modern theories and their use in the development of nursing leadership.

As indicated in the Preface, most of us who experience leadership recognise it when we see it. It has been written about at least since the 16th century, but it remains hard to define and seems to be difficult to produce. Today's achievement-orientated working environments raise questions about the identification of good leadership. How do we recognise it? Can it be learned? Is it always the same? Does someone who leads well in one situation always lead well in a different situation? Are leaders and their skills universally transferable? For example – to elaborate a little on this last question – you may be aware of excellent people who have been highly successful in a particular situation yet fail to transfer those skills and that success to a different environment; perhaps an excellent staff nurse has not fulfilled that perceived potential as a ward sister, an efficient ward sister has crumpled when faced with the wider problems of being a senior nurse, or perhaps even a nurse executive with a glowing reputation in one Trust has never quite moved off the starting blocks in another. These are important questions and important examples, because these situations seem to occur over and over again, and for some reason, even though the answers may be available, we appear to be failing to put the lessons learned into practice.

It was well into the 20th century before social science began to develop theories and undertake the kind of rigorous experiments on group and individual behaviour that would help with the development of valid leadership theories (Adair 1988). Before this, there are only recorded history, anecdote and descriptions of personal experiences to guide and inform any discussion. However, the historical tradition surrounding leadership is very strong, and the historical perspective of leadership is valid for the purpose of this book. In fact, the earliest notions of leadership are still extremely prevalent in our society, regardless of what later research may have shown us. This book starts with arguably the most famous writer on leadership, power and influence – Niccolò Machiavelli.

Machiavelli (1469–1527)

It is well recognised that many aspects of modern life and society had their origins in the Renaissance, the cultural movement of rebirth and modernisation that spread through Europe in the 15th and 16th centuries. In the arts and sciences particularly, a new and enlightened age had begun, but in public life, dynamic changes were taking place, and bitter struggles for power and authority were commonplace. This was the world keenly observed and recorded by Niccolò Machiavelli (1469–1527), a world that was dominated by a new class of politicians and leaders such as Cesare Borgia (1475–1507). While serving as a diplomat for the Republic of Florence, Machiavelli met Borgia and was impressed by his political subtlety and wide-ranging influence.

Probably the earliest well-known writings on leadership and influence are those of Machiavelli, first published in 1532. He used his observations of Cesare Borgia to complete his book *Il Principe* (*The Prince*). So widely known have these writings become that the term 'machiavellian', meaning cunning or duplicitous, has become a part of our language.

The Development of Theories of Leadership

Although his writings are often referred to disparagingly, usually because of a simplistic interpretation of his main theme – the end justifies the means – Machiavelli has much to offer on the subjects of power and influence, both of which are crucial concepts in leadership. Power is an uncomfortable notion for some, but it does have a link with leadership. Leadership is about the ability to cause others to take certain action or to behave in a certain way, about being able to *influence* others. This can be construed as a manifestation of power. Machiavelli identified two key elements in effective leadership:

1. ensuring an adequate and consistent flow of information on important issues
2. behaving respectfully towards those with whom decisions would be jointly taken.

These two elements can be directly related to today's work environments. Ensuring an adequate and consistent flow of information on important issues can be translated virtually unchanged. Today's terms would probably include two-way communication and a logical and planned organisation of the work to be done, that is, being effective. The second element, which recommends behaving respectfully, is more likely to translate into a focus on good working relationships. Maintaining good relationships with decision-making partners – up, across and down the organisation – is crucial. We will explore the importance of relationships in leadership later in the book.

Both being effective and maintaining good relationships occur consistently in modern leadership theory. However, it is Machiavelli's description of the morality, or immorality, of power-seeking for which he is best remembered. Machiavelli's writings are not a scientific study; his conclusions are based on his own experiences and observations of 16th-century politics and power-broking, but his discussions of the tensions that can arise from pursuing public power while maintaining private morality still have an amazing relevance in today's workplace. Dip into a copy of *The Prince* and it is almost guaranteed that, from his descriptions, at least one Prince (or Princess) will be recognised in one's own workplace.

Leader as Hero

The next stop in this trawl through leadership history is the 19th century – quite a big step from Machiavelli back in the 16th. There may well have been discussions and writings on leadership in the intervening centuries, but references have proved difficult to find, even in secondary sources.

In the 19th century, we start to see some evidence of a more systematic approach to the study of leadership, but even so, most writings are based upon leading military and major political figures, thus almost exclusively upon men. Even today, these are the kinds of figure who are mentioned when examples of great leaders are sought. Carlyle (1841 [1907]) concentrated on the qualities of heroic leadership in his discussion of *Heroes and Hero Worship* (although he did, in his title, recognise the symbiotic relationship between leaders and followers). The leader as conquering hero is the traditional way of defining the role and function of the person in charge of the situation – a lone figure leading the way, with a banner and a sword raised high so that the 'troops' can see where to follow (Porter-O'Grady 1992).

Galton (1870), writing in the latter half of the 19th century, also had an heroic vision of leadership, but in addition to this, he believed that leadership was an inherited quality passed from father to son, forming family dynasties of leaders. This reflects the old adage of leaders being born, not made. This early view that leadership ability could depend upon an accident of birth still pervades modern society. The hereditary monarchy system is probably the most obvious example, but some family businesses still operate like this – the eldest child, usually a son, sometimes a daughter, becoming chairperson or chief executive after their father. This often occurs regardless of their suitability or skill actually to do the job. It is still quite common to hear references to individuals being 'born leaders' even though this does not seem like a satisfactory explanation for someone's success. Nevertheless, it continues to be a popular phrase, perpetuating the view that there is something mysterious and indefinable about being a leader.

Webers' Three Bases

In 1947 Weber explored the reasons behind the authority of leaders, and the potential complexity and dynamic nature of effective leadership began to be appreciated. Weber identified three key bases for leadership authority, described by Smith and Peterson (1988) as:

1. the *rational base* – a belief that the prevailing social norm was correct and that those in authority within that social norm had the right to issue orders and commands
2. the *traditional base* – a belief that tradition should steer action, and a belief that those who operate from a traditional power source should be influential
3. the *charismatic base* – a belief in the words, instructions or vision of a person perceived as having a particular sanctity, heroism or exemplary character.

We can still see how these bases for leading and having authority operate in today's environment. Social order, for example, relies heavily upon the rational base. The majority share views about what is appropriate social behaviour and accept the authority figures that arise from those norms – the judiciary, the Church, the government – therefore accepting the checks and balances applied to society through those norms: law and order, statute and regulation, moral codes and so on.

An example of the traditional base can be found in many of our health care environments. Every day, we see examples among our professional medical colleagues of individuals who operate using this base for their authority. Nursing for many years also operated from a traditional base (and in some cases still does). These groups may also be a good example of the charismatic base as well: at least some senior medical and nursing staff operate at a blurred boundary between the traditional and the charismatic base.

The charismatic base can perform on a number of levels. On the one hand, it belongs to the national, or even international, 'guru', the well-known figure who has a ready opinion on every subject and who is usually well respected and listened to by large numbers of people in the same field or with similar interests. On the other, it can also apply to the more local leader who can clearly be seen leading with conviction and who can inspire others to act. This is a brief and probably simplistic description, but charisma will be considered in more detail below.

Even though Weber tried to explore the more complex issues of leadership, the underlying principle continued to be one of traditional, psychosocial expectations – that 'born leaders' will emerge automatically because of the inherent qualities of their mind, spirit and character, which bestow a confident and unquestionable authority upon them. For the first time, however, in the development of leadership theory, Weber had begun to describe how the social or organisational environment could influence leaders and their behaviour.

Discussion Points

Consider individuals in your own environment who might be classed as 'leaders'.

Is any one of them seen as a 'hero(ine)'?

Can you identify people in your own workplace who appear to exercise leadership through:

- a rational base?
- a traditional base?
- a charismatic base?

What is it about their way of working that makes you categorise them into each of these groups?

Throughout the 20th century, the complexities of leadership have continued to be examined and explored by researchers. Smith and Peterson (1988) tell us that, from the 1950s onwards, the importance of the situation in which one was expected to lead became more central to investigations, and the ability to adapt one's responses to different situations became a key feature of effective leadership. At the same time, focusing only on the leader in a group was considered to be too simplistic an approach. Leadership studies began to include the attitudes and responses of the group being led and thus gave a much more rounded picture of how effective leaders achieved their objectives.

In summary, the general literature on leadership up until the last quarter of this century seems to provide us with four major leadership theories, each of which will be explored in more detail in the following chapters:

1. the *personal qualities theory* – that leadership is an innate attribute of the individual's personality
2. the *behavioural style theory* – that leadership is a matter of behaviour and specific activities
3. the *contingency or contextual theory* – that leadership is dependent on and responsive to the situation in which it is required
4. the *group/relationships theory* – that leadership is a collaborative and interactive process.

It would be a mistake, however, to consider leadership as following one of these particular theories in isolation. Effective leaders pick and choose from a range of theories, styles and experiences in order to fit their situation. They are neither rigid in their approach, nor pedantic about the 'right' way to lead.

As this book progresses, you should appreciate the development in thinking from leadership as a personality trait, through leadership as a set of behaviours or as a style, to leadership as a specific reaction to a specific situation. None of these theories on its own can define leadership for us, although they can help us to understand it a little better and, hopefully, harness it for our own use. Leadership, however, is not only about character, skills and situations, but also about relationships and the use of power.

Power

Being an effective leader means that one has influence over certain people – one can cause them to do certain things. Of course, having people do as you tell them does not necessarily make you a leader – you might be a bully, an autocrat or, quite simply, a boss. There are a number of different types of power in organisations. French and Raven (1959, cited in Manfredi 1996) identified five types – expert, referent, legitimate, coercive and reward – but for simplicity, the categories of power put forward by John Adair (1988) in his book *Effective Leadership* will be considered here:

- the power of position
- the power of knowledge
- the power of personality.

Position Power

Position power, as its name implies, stems from one's place, or rank, in the hierarchy and sometimes from the job title. It also includes access to resources – people, equipment and money. This is the power of the boss – anyone who is further up in the hierarchy of the organisation than you are – someone who can hire or fire, give a good or bad reference, structure the working day, notice good (or bad) work and give or take away funding or staff. Hierarchical position always confers a certain degree of power, and the steeper the hierarchy, the more powerful each layer is perceived to be, until one gets to the top. However, those who have travelled through traditional hierarchies will probably already have discovered that position power is not all that it is cracked up to be, particularly if there is no other source of power to enhance it. You have probably heard people saying, 'I could do so much more if I was the ward sister', 'I could do so much more if I had my own unit', 'If only I were a director of nursing, I would change things.' Everybody thinks like this if they work in a hierarchy. The trouble is that these positions entail just as many frustrations and barriers as do those lower down in the system. When progressing through one's career, one needs more than position power to become a leader. A reliance on position power will make it difficult to be accepted as an effective leader – people will do things out of fear rather than because they are inspired by a vision and want to join in

12

with it. Position power can help a leader, but it needs to be matched with other power sources.

Knowledge Power

If someone knows what they are talking about, generally speaking, people will listen. Knowledge power is the stuff of credibility. Credibility will earn respect, respect can give authority, and authority helps by enhancing one's chances of leadership effectiveness. As you progress in your career you will come across quite a few people who are in so-called leadership positions who, sadly, have no credibility. They have no insight into the issues and concerns of the people they are supposed to be leading, and they have no real knowledge of their activities: they have no knowledge power. They can only make things happen through their position power; this is negative and ultimately weak. As observed earlier, this is not what effective leadership needs to be about. *Knowing* the business is one of the most important sources of power in organisations. For nurse leaders it means having a primary knowledge about nurses, about nursing and about the process of nursing as it happens to the patients in their care. To be in a senior position in health care, or to be an executive nurse, a secondary knowledge about finance, politics and people, among other things, is also needed. You do not need to know everything about everything; but you do need to know enough to be credible with people outside your own professional group.

If you are knowledgeable then you may be able to lead without any formal position power at all. People will look to you for direction because you 'talk a lot of sense', or you 'talk their language'. The phrase 'getting the opinion leaders on board in an organisation', means getting the support of the informal leaders – the people with knowledge power who can influence their colleagues and peers. Influencing through knowledge is a very strong type of power.

Personality Power and Charisma

This is where we start to talk about 'charisma', found in those people referred to as 'born leaders'. These are the motivational speakers, people who are out in front telling you what they believe in and what you should believe in. They touch you because they share your experiences and seem to know just how you are feeling. They inspire you to greater determination and self-help. Individuals with personality power can be a long way ahead in the leadership stakes.

But personality power is easy to abuse; it is easy to become fond of the sound of one's own voice and forget to keep knowledge up to date. It is easy to be seduced by professional media attention and become all personality with no position and precious little knowledge of the real world. Credibility will disappear eventually. Personality power can also be abused if it is used only to serve the interests of the powerful rather than to meet the needs of the followers. Think, for example, of some of the religious or spiritual type of personality cults where the needs of individuals are completely subjugated by the desires of their leader. This is an extreme example, but there is a relatively common type of personality power that is mostly self-interested, and this can be just as negative and weak as relying only on position.

While we are discussing personality power, we should spend some time considering the notion of charisma. Because charisma is a type of personality power, it is a very real source of influence. It is a tangible asset in the leadership skills repertoire that can be learned and used when the situation demands. It seems odd to think of charisma as a skill that can be switched on and off at will, but I believe it can be used in this way. Obviously some people will be better at it than others, but the same is true of any other skill that it is possible to learn. For example, I can be a charismatic speaker when I think my audience needs rousing and motivating. But if I spoke to people in charismatic mode all the time, then they might well get bored. It would not be appropriate for every situation. Some people can be incredibly charming when they need to be, when they need allegiance or support, but they can switch that charm off as easily as they seem to switch it on. This is not as deceitful as you might think –

14

charisma is a legitimate technique that can be chosen in the same way that one chooses to use other skills.

Davidhizar (1993) has analysed charisma and sees it as an important characteristic that can be useful for leaders who want to motivate through positive relationships rather than by utilising controlling or authoritarian-type approaches. She has identified a number of elements that she believes demonstrate the concept of charisma:

- being able to communicate positive self-esteem
- focusing on people
- having a clear vision
- promoting the vision to others
- implementing the vision.

Leaders who use charisma feel good about themselves and about other people. They are interested in people and encourage the group to accomplish the task, rather than focusing on the task itself. They know where they are going and where they want to take others. They are able to articulate that future in a way that motivates and encourages others, and they are able to get the job done together.

A charismatic personality can turn good managers into powerful leaders. However, relying on the power of personality is incredibly hard work. Having to make up for a lack of position power and a lack of resources by sheer force of personality will lead to burn-out in no time. Be wary of any job description or advertisement that talks about influencing and motivating but gives no indication of resources or positional authority – it will probably wear you out! Having said that, in the current climate of devolved management responsibilities, most NHS Trust nurse executives have to rely on a mix of knowledge, personality and charisma to get their work done. Traditional position power, in terms of line authority, is seldom available to them. It may be that there is a relationship between the stresses of relying on personality and knowledge and the fact that nurse executives stay for only an average of 2.8 years in post (Ball 1996). This is worth considering if you have aspirations to lead at that level of the service.

Power versus Leadership

If one of the purposes of this book is to help promote a better understanding of leadership, although it is important to understand about power and how it works, it is equally important to understand the differences between power and leadership. Power, like leadership, is a relationship between leaders and followers, both involving motivation, resources and influence (Trofino 1993). When leaders influence their followers' behaviour in order to meet their own goals, what they are doing is exercising power. If, when they are influencing to achieve goals, leaders also manage to satisfy the motives and needs of their followers, they are exercising leadership. The crux of the matter is in that relationship with followers and whether it is passive or collaborative. The importance of relationships is a continuous theme in leadership and will be discussed at various points in later chapters.

This brief tour through the main developments in leadership research and theory, and the main sources of power in organisations, completes this introduction. The next chapter will look more closely at the three main interpretations of leadership:

1. as a personal quality
2. as a behavioural style
3. as a contingent or contextual response.

Discussion Points

Consider your own notions of power. What makes a person powerful in your eyes?

Consider the people who are perceived as powerful in your workplace. Who are they? What makes them powerful? Can you identify why they may be viewed as being powerful using the information from this chapter?

What sort of power do you think that you have in your role?

References

References marked * are from a secondary source: Smith P and Peterson M (1988) *Leadership, Organisations and Culture*. Sage. London.

Adair J (1988) *Effective Leadership*. Pan. London.
Ball J (1996) *Nurse Executive Pay – A Survey for the Royal College of Nursing*. RCN. London.
*Carlyle T (1841 [1907]) *Heroes and Hero Worship*. Adams. Boston.
Davidhizar A (1993) Leading with charisma. *Journal of Advanced Nursing*. 18: 675–9.
*Galton F (1870) *Hereditary Genius*. Appleton. New York.
Machiavelli N (1532). *Il Principe*. Translated by Bondanella P and Musa M (1984) as *The Prince*. Oxford University Press. Oxford.
Manfredi C (1996) A descriptive study of nurse managers and leadership. *Western Journal of Nursing Research*. 18(3): 314–29.
Porter-O'Grady T (1992) Transformational leadership in an age of chaos. *Nursing Administration Quarterly*. 17(1): 17–24.
Trofino J (1993) Transformational leadership: the catalyst for successful change. *International Nursing Review*. 40(6): 179–82, 187.
*Weber M (1947) *The Theory of Economic and Social Organisation*. Translated by Henderson AM and Parsons T. Free Press. New York.

Chapter 2 Interpretations of Leadership

This chapter discusses the three main interpretations of leadership – as a personal quality, as a behavioural style and as a contingent approach – by reviewing the commonly cited literature on these three elements. In a book of this type, full and detailed descriptions are obviously not appropriate, but additional reading can be found in the references at the end of this chapter. In reviewing the development of leadership theories, I have tried to choose those studies which have been considered to be important in their time and which have contributed to the development of thinking. It is prudent, however, in these early chapters to bear in mind that times change and that these older studies should be considered for their effect in their own historical context and how they influenced thinking, as well as for their continuing application and relevance in today's environment.

Leadership as a Personal Quality

Whenever I discuss leadership with a group, or ask nurses to say what they think leadership is, the initial response is usually a list of personal traits or qualities. People talk about 'integrity', 'the ability to work hard', 'lateral thinking', 'enthusiasm', 'the ability to make decisions' and 'self-confidence' among others. Since the 1930s, lists of leadership qualities have appeared regularly in the literature. But is effective leadership really that simple? For example, we all know people who are brilliant lateral thinkers but we could not say that they are leaders; likewise, some confident people and good decision-makers do not demonstrate what can be recognised as leadership. Nonetheless, leadership as an aggregation of personal traits is an interesting concept and should be briefly explored.

There have been a great many studies examining personal traits and their links with leadership and leadership potential. Stogdill (1948) and Mann (1959) located between them 179 studies of this type, and, following their reviews, both came to the conclusion that personal traits account for only a small proportion of variance in leadership behaviour. Mann's work actually showed a low correlation between leadership and personal traits. However, we should not dismiss personal traits as an indicator of leadership potential on the basis of these findings but should at least find out a little more about these studies. Most of the studies that Stogdill and Mann reviewed were concerned with the behaviour of children or students in informal environments. In spite of this limitation, these studies are often discussed and related to adult behaviour in structured work settings, where the influence of the environment and other factors may be very different. In addition to this, very few of these studies looked at the effectiveness of the leader – did the person identified as the leader get the job done? And is 'getting the job done' a reasonable indicator of leadership effectiveness anyway?

In 1974 Stogdill reviewed a further 163 studies linking personal qualities and leadership that had been published since his earlier review of 1948. These included studies of effective leadership and also studies of adults in structured work settings. This time, Stogdill came to the conclusion that his earlier work had underestimated the influence of personal qualities on leadership and they should, after all, be considered as factors contributing to effective leadership. He reported several personal characteristics that were frequently linked to leadership, including:

- activity level
- intelligence
- dominance
- self-confidence
- drive for achievement
- interpersonal skills.

It is worth pausing here to reflect on Stogdill's list of characteristics. They may well have been appropriate in 1974, but are they all appropriate in today's working environments and organisational cultures?

Discussion Points

What do you think about the above list in relation to leadership?

Would you consider some of these traits to be more or less significant today than in the 1970s?

Which of those traits would you include in a list of your own? Which would you leave out? Why?

If we think about Stogdill's list, we can see that some of these characteristics are actually skills or attributes rather than facets of someone's personality. Drawing upon my own experience when discussing the necessary attributes of an effective leader with nurses, other factors, such as good communication skills, resilience under pressure and the ability to deal with uncertainty, start to appear. If we then link effective leadership to managerial success, even more factors present themselves. For example, Miner (1978) identified a desire for power, competition with peers and positive attitudes to authority as success factors. Later work by Miner and Crane (1981) emphasised the desire for power as being particularly important in predicting success. This notion of 'desire for power' is an intriguing point and one of the reasons why the general literature on leadership may not be completely transferable to nursing; in personal discussions with nurses, I have found that a *desire* for power is rarely mentioned as a motivating factor for nurse leaders, nor is competitiveness. In fact, nurse leaders tend, on the whole, to be rather uncomfortable with the notions of both power and competitiveness. Power is mentioned frequently, however, but in the context of being able to *use* power positively. For many nurse leaders, it seems to be the constructive *use* of power that is important rather than the *desire* for power. This is a subtle difference but a quite significant one in terms of motivation – one for the researchers to investigate.

The link with managerial success brings into play a completely different collection of characteristics, but we need to consider whether managerial success is the same as effective leadership. It appears not to be, for the following reasons.

Rost (1994) explains that management is located within an organisation – it is concerned with maintaining the organisation and reaching the stated goals of that organisation. Managers take on the responsibility of directing the work of others, usually subordinates, and of making decisions on behalf of others. They also usually have and exercise formal organisational authority, involving themselves in ensuring the competence and development of subordinates and acting as role models for aspiring managers. Leadership does not have to be about organisations. It can take place anywhere, in any situation where people are required to work together to achieve change. Its emphasis is on the shared achievement of mutual goals rather than the acceptance of one person's responsibility for a stated outcome achieved through others. Leadership also emphasises the promotion of shared values and desire for change. It is facilitative rather than directive, mutual rather than authoritative, empowering rather than coercive. Leadership nurtures and encourages the personal growth of others while achieving mutual objectives.

Management and leadership can have similar ends but are very different means. They are often confused, being talked of in the same terms. Unfortunately, by not properly separating out the differences, we only prolong the time it will take for nursing appropriately to prepare effective leaders for the future. Teaching management skills will not necessarily produce leaders or even encourage leadership skills. Measures of success are important to the leadership debate, and managerial success may be one factor – but it is only one. We need criteria that tell us how to recognise leadership. If we are not sure of the particular criteria that tell us what leadership is, it is going to be almost impossible to monitor it, measure it or teach it. During the final drafting of this book, I discovered the work of Professor J. C. Rost, who clarifies this 'leadership versus management' question extremely well (Rost 1994). Some of his views will be explored later in the book.

In more scientific arenas, the 'leadership as personal quality' approach is disliked because it is so subjective. Can it really be true that the person who emerges as a leader in a group does so only because he or she possesses certain personal characteristics, that leadership is not learned but is a latent quality in certain personality types? The personal quality approach is debatable as a stand-alone theory but is still able to contribute to this debate. Charismatic leadership is certainly well recognised, and, as we have already discussed, is connected to personality.

Discussion Points

What are the personal qualities that you expect to find in a leader?

Can someone be a leader if he or she does not possess these personal qualities?

Can you think of someone who is a leader and who does not possess these personal qualities?

Consider someone whom you respect as a leader. List the things about that person that make them a leader. Look at your list and see how many items on it are personal qualities.

Leadership as a Behavioural Style

So far, we have looked at defining leadership as an innate personal quality, a quality that makes it acceptable, even desirable, to have influence over others, a quality ensuring that others respond effectively. These views have become modified over a period of time. The set of behaviours, or traits – for example confidence, dominance, intelligence and so on – that were identified as being related to leadership were relatively well accepted into the early part of the 20th century. After the 1930s, however, it was proposed that they were not actually inherent in the person but were styles of behaviour that were consciously enacted – they were styles that could be taught – and learned. This was a big step forward, in terms of equal opportunities, if nothing else.

The most well-known study of different leadership styles is probably that of Lewin *et al.* (1939), which examined the effects of leadership styles in boys clubs in the USA. The researchers compared democratic and autocratic leadership styles and reported a more favourable response to the democratic than the autocratic style. Within this context, democratic refers to a style which encourages participation in decision-making by those being led, and autocratic to situations in which decisions were made by leaders and imposed upon those being led without discussion between the parties concerned. However, a 'favourable response' seems to depend upon the criteria used to define what constitutes 'favourable'. For example, morale was good when a democratic style was used, but productivity was improved with an autocratic style.

This study was influential in America and the UK during the Second World War, but replication studies carried out since then in other cultures have questioned the findings. For example, Japanese researchers found that democracy worked if the task was easy, but autocracy was more effective when the task was difficult. In addition, researchers in India found autocracy to be more effective whatever the situation or complexity of the task. It appears that a style effective in Western cultures is not necessarily transferable to others. These lessons about effectiveness can be applied not only to 'culture' in an ethnic context, but also to organisational culture, something that will be considered below.

In the 1950s, researchers began to consider the existing style of leaders who were well established in their positions in organisations. For the first time, they developed questionnaires reflecting the perceptions of behaviour and effectiveness of both the leader and the group being led. As a result of this development, Stogdill and Coons (1957) concluded that leadership styles vary in two areas: 'consideration' and 'initiating structure'. In simple terms, this means that a good leader would not only be considerate to others, but also provide appropriate structures to enable the task to be completed.

Throughout the 1960s and 70s, leadership style measurement scales became very popular, and through a wide range of studies, it became clear that the relationship between style and performance (defined as effectiveness in getting the job done) was extremely variable. As a result of these studies, important connections were being made between leadership, the environment and the ability to adapt one's approach to the situation. A new theory was emerging: it seemed that although the average person in a leadership position exceeded the average member of the group in a number of personal characteristics, the actual *skills* needed were determined to a large extent by the requirements of the situation in which the leader was trying to function (Smith and Peterson 1988). Because the results of these studies varied so widely, researchers began to explore other avenues. Research into leadership style seemed to be failing to provide generalisable conclusions: although styles could be identified relatively easily, their effectiveness was not as predictable. This variability in result, even when similar or identical styles were used, led to a complete reconceptualisation of leadership theory.

When I discuss leadership styles with nurses in workshops, they talk about democracy, fairness, leading by example (particularly in clinical leadership positions), enabling, empowering – all good, positive stuff. When they are asked to think about a particularly difficult task that they had to achieve and how their 'leader' behaved in those circumstances, quite a different set of words come out – giving clear direction, leading from the front, 'taking' the group where they needed to go. These descriptions often related to the same person who had previously been described as democratic, empowering and so on. Yet this change in behaviour did not arouse any hostility or reluctance but was instead seen as being appropriate to the situation. This notion of fitting a leadership style to the situation at hand led to the development of contingency theories.

Discussion Points

Describe the way in which you would expect an autocratic leader to behave. What are the advantages and disadvantages of working in this way?

Describe the way in which you would expect a democratic leader to behave. What are the advantages and disadvantages of working in this way?

Do you think that it is possible to be both democratic and autocratic?

Leadership as a Contingency Approach

The third development around the concept of leadership was the emergence of a theory claiming that any one style of leadership is contingent upon the environment within which the leader is operating. It seems that the emergence of leaders, and the characteristics that they display, are a direct result of the specific situation and will vary according to that situation. This led the way to the more modern view that different organisational settings require different concepts or styles of leadership. This takes us back to our thoughts in the previous few pages that leadership style may need to alter in order to be effective in different cultures.

One of the earliest contingency theories of leadership effectiveness appears to be that of Fiedler (1967). Fiedler proposed that people became leaders not just because of their attributes or personalities, but also because of various situational factors and interactions between the leader and group members. Fiedler distinguishes between task-orientated leaders and relationship-orientated leaders, suggesting that these styles alter according to what he calls 'situational favorability'. He maintains that situations will allow varying levels of leader influence depending upon three factors:

1. the quality of the relationship with subordinates
2. the leader's formal position in the organisation
3. the degree of task structure.

Fiedler claims that, in highly unfavourable situations where there is poor position power, unclear tasks and poor relationships, a task-orientated leader will bring structure and direction and will gain authority from taking such actions. Fiedler also suggests that where the environment is highly favourable – with high position power, good relationships and so on – the task-orientated leader can be equally successful. However, in situations that are neither highly favourable nor highly unfavourable, the relationship-orientated leader is more likely to succeed. Looking back to the previous chapter, this seems to advocate a mix of charismatic power and positional power, together with some management skills. Looking forward, these concepts will reappear below when we discuss the modern theories of transformational and transactional leadership styles.

This situational approach to leadership introduced the notion of flexible and varying leadership responses. The situation will determine not only the leader, but also the leadership strategy that should be adopted. 'Different strokes for different folks' is a truism that seems to apply to leadership approaches. Fiedler's theory, however, still does to some extent relate to personality traits. There are other contingency models that do not relate so closely to concepts of personality.

Leadership research became more and more complex, reflecting the nature of leadership itself through the 1970s and 80s. The influence of motivation was recognised, and 'path-goal' theory was developed. The most commonly cited path-goal theory is Victor Vroom's work from 1964. In simple terms, path-goal theory makes two main assertions. In order for groups to do what leaders want them to, leaders must ensure:

- that group members know how to accomplish goals
- that group members achieve their personal goals in the process.

That is, group members have to be competent to do what is being asked of them, and there has to be something in it for them.

In order to achieve these two key factors, House and Dressler (1974) and House and Mitchell (1974) identified four possible leadership styles that may be useful:

1. *instrumental* – directive, with clear instructions – Caroline
2. *supportive* – facilitative, encouraging others to solve their own problems – Ali
3. *participative* – working with group members, offering advice and joining in decision-making – Me
4. *achievement-orientated* – concentrating on the task and the outcome.

When deciding which of these four styles to use, leaders need to consider the personal characteristics of the group they are trying to lead and the environment in which they work. This

26

notion of *choosing* a leadership style becomes an obvious skill requirement once leadership is accepted to be about relationships and working together.

Heller and Wilpert (1981) claimed that leadership style was significantly influenced by the nature of the decision to be made and found that successful leaders related their style to much broader environmental factors than just the specific task in hand. Still more complex contingency theories continued to develop. The anticipated response of the group being led began to be considered, this eventually becoming a key feature in choosing a leadership style.

As these theories developed, first with their emphasis on the situation, and later with their emphasis on all the players involved rather than just the leader, so the importance of relationships in leadership came to the fore. This will be discussed in Chapter 3.

Discussion Points

Consider a scenario from your own workplace in which you or a colleague exercised leadership. Was your/their approach the same from the beginning to the end of the situation? Break the scenario down into stages – can you identify whether the leader was more directive at a particular stage, or more facilitative at another? Describe these differences and what prompted the change of style, if any occurred.

If there were no differences, do you think that a more flexible approach might have helped? If not, what was it about the situation that made one approach more reasonable than any other?

References

References marked * are from a secondary source: Smith P and Peterson M (1988) *Leadership, Organisations and Culture*. Sage. London. This provides a very comprehensive review of the general literature relating to leadership.

Fiedler FE (1967) *A Contingency Theory of Leadership and Effectiveness*. McGraw-Hill. London.

Heller A and Wilpert A (1981) *Competence and Power in Managerial Decision Making*. John Wiley. Chichester.

*House RJ and Dressler G (1974) The path-goal theory of leadership – some *post hoc* and *a priori* tests. *Contingency Approaches to Leadership*. Southern Illinois University Press.

*House RJ and Mitchell TR (1974) The path-goal theory of leadership. *Journal of Contemporary Business*. **3**: 31–97.

*Lewin K, Lippitt R and White RK (1939) Patterns of aggressive behaviour in experimentally created social climates. *Journal of Social Psychology*. **10**: 271–99.

*Mann RD (1959) A review of the relationships between personality and performance in small groups. *Psychological Bulletin*. **56**: 241–70.

*Miner JB (1978) Twenty years research on role motivation theory of management effectiveness. *Personnel Psychology*. **31**: 739–60.

*Miner JB and Crane DP (1981) Motivation to manage and the manifestation of a managerial orientation in career planning. *Academy of Management Journal*. **24**: 626–33.

Rost JC (1994) Leadership: a new conception. *Holistic Nursing Practice*. **9**(1): 1–8.

*Stogdill RM (1948) Personal factors associated with leadership: a survey of the literature. *Journal of Psychology*, **25**: 35–71.

*Stogdill RM (1974) *A Handbook of Leadership*. Free Press. New York.

*Stogdill RM and Coons AE (eds) (1957) *Leader Behaviour: Its Description and Measurement*. Bureau of Business Research. Ohio State University.

Vroom V (1964) *Work and Motivation*. John Wiley. London.

Chapter 3 Interpersonal Skills and Leadership

This chapter will discuss the importance of interpersonal skills and the relationship between the leaders and those being led. The discussion will again take the form of a review of the literature relating to leadership.

Leadership and Relationships

As leadership theory continued to develop, so the role of those being led began to become more important. The relationship between leaders and their followers began to be explored, and the crucial role that leaders play in bringing together people from different levels within the organisation was recognised. As long ago as 1961, Likert was describing the leader as the 'linkpin', forming a connection with the group of followers that was fundamental to their being able to function successfully.

However, it is not only the leader/follower relationship that makes a difference: there is also a whole range of interpersonal connections that seem to have an effect. For example, there are studies cited in Smith and Peterson (1988) showing that leaders will be more influential with their followers if they demonstrate good relationships with their own boss. Therefore, it seems that the people you want to lead may well judge your credibility to do so on the basis of the quality of your working relationships with your own leaders. They may also judge your approach to providing leadership and decide their reactions according to how appropriate they feel that approach is to the situation at hand.

This makes the whole process of leadership much more complex and brings in a whole new range of considerations for aspiring leaders. It also brings us back to the concept of power, as this recognition of the actions and reactions of followers creates a definite shift in the traditional power relationship between leaders and followers. We see the development of a much more equal distribution of power between the group and the leader, which is a quite different view from that of the traditional and historical notions of leadership. It also appears that there is a need for collective understanding in order to facilitate effective leadership and reduce role conflict. Collective understanding refers to the circumstance whereby both leader and followers have a shared view of the task in hand or the way forward. Thinking about a collective understanding of situations means that we will have to consider the organisational culture in which we are working when we consider which approach to leadership to adopt.

Organisational Culture

The subject of organisational culture crops up a great deal in the literature on leadership, management and organisational development. It seems to be a crucial factor in any activity or strategy that involves change, particularly in any action to implement change. It is often cited as the motivator for change; for example, the prevailing organisational culture may not lend itself to the direction in which an organisation needs to go in order to survive. It is also often cited as a reason for failure, again because the prevailing organisational culture would not allow the activities necessary to bring about a change.

All organisations have their own ways of going about their everyday business, things that work for them and things that do not (Belasco 1990); it is these unspoken and unwritten processes that make up their organisational culture. Schein (1985) defines organisational culture as the set of assumptions that are recognised and accepted within an organisation in order to enable collective understanding to occur – when people interpret things in the same way and share the same hopes, fears and expectations. These are the assumptions about where power and influence lie in the organisation, about what really motivates people, about how the organisation thinks and reacts and about the kinds of approach that might encourage it to change. Collective understanding, and the organisational culture that arises from it, can be an amazingly positive experience and a powerful force for improvement and change; conversely, it can be a destructive and restraining factor.

Organisational culture is frequently further complicated by the various group values, desires, philosophies and relationships within it. Getting a whole organisation, with all its disparate internal groups, to share the same values, desires and objectives is extremely difficult. Most organisational cultures are the result of past experience, traditional thinking and working patterns, and the responses of people to their working relationships. Large and complex organisations such as NHS Trusts will often have a variety of group cultures operating within them, although there is usually a prevailing culture that pervades the organisation as a whole and has been formed by past experience, relationships and group expectations based upon these.

Being a leader nearly always means tackling organisational culture change at some point, or at least working with or around particular cultures. It is important for leaders to remember that understanding the culture in which they work is vital. They often have to begin to change the prevailing culture in order for people to see the need or want to change anything else.

People working in organisations are sensitive to the signals emanating from their particular organisation. These signals can come from different parts of the organisation, for example from pay and reward strategies or from promotion patterns, but the signals are strongest when they come from what the mass of the organisation thinks is 'the done thing'. This is the organisational culture at work. Organisational culture is intangible but is very much there, and the people who work in the organisation know and understand it very well indeed. That is why newcomers can be at such a disadvantage on first joining an organisation: it takes a little while to learn the signals and to respond to them in the expected way in order to 'fit' into the organisation. The rules inherent in this informal organisational culture can carry more weight than all the systems, policies and procedures that can be produced, because adherence to these unspoken rules often defines 'belonging' to or acceptance within the organisation.

Johnson and Scholes (1993) claim that organisational culture can be broken down into the following elements:

- *control systems* – which aspects of the organisation are most closely monitored, promoted or emphasised?
- *power structures* – what are the underlying beliefs of the most powerful people in the organisation?
- *stories* – what do people gossip about, whom do they talk about, how do they describe the organisation?
- *symbols* – who has the biggest office, who wears a uniform, is there an internal 'language'?
- *organisational structure* – is it flat or steep? Is there a strict hierarchy or a matrix?
- *rituals and routines* – what things are taken for granted? Are there longstanding meetings and committees? Are certain activities sacrosanct?

If you can analyse your own organisation by trying to answer those questions, you will probably have a pretty good idea of the prevailing organisational culture within which you are working. You will be able to use this knowledge to consider appropriate strategies for leading within that culture, thus increasing the chances of success if change is needed.

Discussion Points

Can you describe the culture of the organisation in which you work?

What are its particular rituals and routines?

Would you describe the culture as mainly positive or mainly negative?

Can you identify anyone within your organisation who very obviously does not 'fit' with the prevailing culture? What is it about this person that makes you identify them like this?

What sort of leadership approaches do you think would be best suited to your organisation?

Understanding organisational culture and group expectations is another element of the leadership portfolio, and it will mean that you understand the standard ways in which things happen – or do not happen – in your organisation.

Groups and Group Relationships

All leaders will need to work with a group or groups of other people, and we have already discussed the influence that groups can have and how crucial a component of leadership being able to work with this influence can be. However, if the group is so important, how does the notion of 'leader' fit in with the group or relationships approach, particularly if the accepted definition of a group is a number of equals, or at least like-minded individuals, working together on a shared objective? In this instance, having an individual who is called a leader does not seem to be at all appropriate, and neither does using the term 'follower'.

We could start by not interpreting the term 'group' as only meaning a number of individuals gathered together to complete a task. In reality, people in leadership positions will be required to work in and around a number of groups during the course of their work. These may be groups of subordinates, groups of peers, groups brought together to achieve a specific function and so on. In reality, the group, when seen in relation to the leader, actually consists of a wide range of contacts and individuals who are not necessarily a cohesive unit.

Leaders do not usually limit their attention to just one group. When leaders are observed, they have been found to spend as much, if not more, time on relationships with their peers and colleagues as they do on relationships with their subordinates and superiors. In a review of the literature by Sayles (1964), the conclusion was drawn that effective leaders do not simply cultivate good relationships higher up and lower down the organisation, but also spend much time building and maintaining a whole set of complex and interconnected relationships across, and sometimes beyond, the whole organisation. Leaders do not necessarily see themselves as, or behave as if they are, 'in charge' of groups. Their relationships cross boundaries of role and position, and they behave in a collaborative way. An integrated matrix of relationships appears to be crucial to the effectiveness of the leader. A colleague and friend of mine – a highly respected and influential nurse leader – once described her working methods to me as 'basket-weaving my way through the organisation', a perfect description of how one needs to make contact with and interrelate with many other individuals and groups.

Discussion Points

Think of someone you consider to be a good leader. How do they relate to people?

Are their relationships generally constructive and positive?

Do they have equally good relationships with subordinates, peers and superiors?

Is there any difference in their behaviour with each of these groups?

Think of a leader whom you respect and admire. What is it about them that makes you want to 'follow'?

Facilitator versus Leader?

In group work, it currently seems that identifying someone called a 'group leader' is less popular and that working groups are more likely to have a 'facilitator' to help them undertake their work. I have been asked on a number of occasions whether facilitators are the same as leaders.

According to Heron (1979), a good facilitator needs to have an awareness of how groups work – their 'dynamics'. This includes the underlying behaviour of individual members as well as the actual content of discussion. Facilitators need to have an understanding of when a particular function or intervention is required and to have the skills to intervene effectively, that is, to cause the group to respond or change course. Causing a group to respond sounds like a leadership function, so perhaps facilitation and leadership do overlap. Helping people to make decisions, encouraging problem-solving, diffusing conflict, changing direction – these are all skills expected from a facilitator and a leader. According to the literature we have briefly reviewed so far, a facilitator must be acceptable and credible to the group, as must a leader. So does being a good facilitator make you a leader? In one way, it does. Are the terms 'leader' and 'facilitator' interchangeable? In certain circumstances, they could perhaps be. A good facilitator is utilising skills associated with leadership when working with the group. However, facilitation is not all that there is to leadership, even though effective facilitation is one way of demonstrating leadership.

Discussion Points

Read about facilitation skills. List the main ones. Go back to the descriptions of leadership skills that you made earlier. How many of the skills appear on both lists?

Can you identify what the main differences between a facilitator and a leader might be? (It might be helpful to consider their functions.)

Are the differences to do with behaviour or with the context of the situation?

How groups, and individuals, react to leaders is of fundamental importance. Relationships are crucial to leadership effectiveness. In fact, Rost (1994) states that leadership *is* relationships. Just stop and think about it for a moment – if no-one is going along with you, can you really consider yourself to be a leader?

Putting it Together

The leadership theories mentioned in these three chapters – personal qualities, behavioural style, contingency and group/relationships – are not alternative approaches; instead they should be seen as complementary. A truly comprehensive approach to leadership should contain all the major factors known to be involved –

the personality of the leader, the followers and their attitudes, needs and problems, the group itself and the situation. Smith and Peterson (1988) have emphasised that effective leadership is a matter not of developing a certain style but of learning how to choose the right approach in order to obtain maximum benefit. Even this is not as straightforward as it first appears. Some leaders may well have all the skills and attributes, even the charismatic features, that enable them to influence and negotiate, but they may not have access to the resources that allow them to make really appropriate decisions, particularly if they are inexperienced. Resources include, for example, wide networks, access to expert advice and access to sources of information. A wide and varied resource base provides leaders with the maximum amount of information to help them to make choices about appropriate strategies.

Out in the real world, leaders have to pick their way between conflicting demands, conflicting value sets, lobbying and pressure groups and so on, making choices about which strategies or specific behaviours will give them the best result. If they have been able to integrate themselves into a particular culture (where they understand the underpinning philosophy and values of an organisation), this may well help, but prevailing organisational culture can, on the other hand, often produce constraint rather than choice. It is in these situations that experience can be of real value.

References

Belasco J (1990) *Teaching the Elephant to Dance*. Hutchinson Business Books. London.
Heron J (1979) *The Facilitator's Handbook*. Kogan Page. London.
Johnson G and Scholes K (1993) *Exploring Corporate Strategy*. Prentice-Hall. London.
Likert R (1961) *New Patterns of Management*. McGraw-Hill. London.
Rost JC (1994) Leadership: a new conception. *Holistic Nursing Practice*. 9(1): 1–8.
Sayles SR (1964) *Managerial Behaviour*. McGraw-Hill. London.
Schein EH (1985) *Organisational Culture and Leadership – A Dynamic View*. Jossey Bass. London.
Smith P and Peterson M (1988) *Leadership, Organisations and Culture*. Sage. London.

Summary and Conclusion to Chapters 1–3

The general literature on leadership appears to provide us with four major leadership theories:

1. the personal qualities theory
2. the behavioural style theory
3. the contingency theory
4. the group/relationships theory.

Recent literature seems to advise us that the most effective approach is probably a combination of all four of these theories. This, together with the ability to make critical choices, seems most likely to lead to success.

In the late 1980s and early 1990s, there certainly appears to have been a resurgence of the 'personality/qualities' theory, with many leadership gurus describing 'their' way. Recent popular literature on leadership also seems to stress the evangelical and the charismatic. Think of people like Tom Peters of *Thriving on Chaos* and *In Search of Excellence* fame, John Harvey-Jones when he is *Troubleshooting*, or Charles Handy with his books of mass popular appeal. These are all leaders of a sort because they can affect the behaviour of others: they have influence. Consider such recent political figures as Margaret Thatcher and John Major, or Tony Blair and the late John Smith – who appealed most to their respective audiences? How about Richard Branson or Anita Roddick? In recent times, charismatic or personality-based leadership remains as popular and attractive as ever in all kinds of fields, regardless of any research evidence that may question its validity.

In addition to the strength of charisma, we know that effective leadership seems to require the ability to *choose* appropriate strategies and to *implement* them successfully, influencing other interested parties in a positive way. Charles Handy, mentioned above and one of the most popular and well-respected management and leadership development thinkers of recent times, maintains that successful organisations need 'leadership of ideas, not of personality', people who can think about today's problems in a new and different way, so that they cease to be problems for the future. Handy (1990) talks about the 'post-heroic' leader. He defines the heroic leader as a know-all, do-all, solve-every-problem-for-you type that is no longer appropriate and compares him with the post-heroic leader who asks how a problem might be solved in a way that develops other people's capacity to handle it. It seems that the post-heroic leader is not in it for the personal acclaim, or the feeling of success, but for the sense of gratification that comes from having helped others to achieve success (Mant 1985). Handy uses the term 'transformational' to describe this theory of leadership.

Transformational leadership was first identified by James MacDonald Burns (1978) and further refined by Tichy and Devanna (1986). This approach to leadership concentrates on the ability to influence situations or people by affecting their ways of thinking, even affecting their underlying values. This is usually juxtaposed with the 'transactional' approach, which is more concerned with doing and putting things right for others. The notion of transformational leadership is such a popular concept that it will be discussed in more detail when we move on to leadership in nursing in Chapter 4.

References

Burns JM (1978) *Leadership*. Harper & Row. New York.
Handy C (1990) *The Age of Unreason*. Arrow. London.
Mant A (1985) *Leaders We Deserve*. Martin Robertson. London.
Tichy NM and Devanna MA (1986) The transformational leader. *Training and Development Journal*. **40**(7): 27–32.

Further Reading on Group Work

Heron J (1979) *The Facilitator's Handbook*. Kogan Page. London.
Hinshelwood RD (1987) *What Happens in Groups*. Free Association Books. London.
Bolman L (1976) Group leader effectiveness. In Cooper C (ed.) *Developing Social Skills in Managers*. Macmillan. London.

Chapter 4 Leadership in Nursing

The notion of leadership in nursing has, until fairly recently, been inadequately explored. There is very little research into nursing leadership in the UK dating from before 1980, but interest and subsequent publications are now increasing, and since the 1980s there has been considerable debate and discussion. The growing interest is closely linked to the political and organisational changes and influences that have affected nurses and nursing management over the past 30 years or so in the UK, and while leadership and management are recognised as two separate issues, changes in one are likely to have affected the other. It is thus difficult to discuss leadership in nursing without placing it in its historical, political and managerial context.

In the Preface to this book, I remarked upon how nurses continually search for better or different leadership, apparently considering the existing leadership to be in some way inadequate. It has to be agreed that the direction of nursing, both nationally and locally, sometimes seems to be hard to follow. We have blamed our leaders over the years for a multitude of dissatisfactions – clinical grading, education changes, crises in recruitment and retention, inadequate pay and poor conditions, lack of power. Nursing undoubtedly suffers, or has suffered, from all of these things and more, but an examination of the history and politics of the situation may well help us to understand better why nursing seems to have some difficulty in controlling its own destiny. In order to hold a leadership role in nursing, it is important to understand its prevailing environment and how the past has influenced and shaped the present.

History and Politics

The history of nursing is a fascinating subject in its own right, and only the key milestones during its recent history can be highlighted here. For those wishing to explore nursing's history in more depth, the reference section of this chapter provides more information.

Nursing has been called the oldest of the arts and the youngest of the professions (Donahue 1985). It began as the role of the mother nourishing infants and nurturing young children, and slowly developed to encompass care of the sick, the aged, the helpless and the infirm. At first, this care was confined within the immediate family, but it then began to broaden into providing a service outside the home. Its driving forces at this time were love, humanitarianism and altruism. Over a period of time, it became apparent that love and caring alone could not ensure health or overcome disease. The development of nursing needed additional elements – skill, expertise and knowledge. The science, spirit and skill of nursing were thus beginning to develop (Stewart 1918, 1921).

In its early years, nursing had a primarily religious background, arising from the Christian teachings of love, brotherhood and service to others. Altruism was interpreted as a disinterested service to humanity, devotion to others without thought of reward, done for the love of God. From this concept of Christian altruism developed the orders of men and women in the early church who cared for the sick and weak. This spiritual period of nursing's history is where the notion of the nurses' 'calling' originated.

In the Middle Ages, the concept of the holy war and the increasing religious fervour that fuelled the Crusades led to the development of military nursing orders, the religious military such as the Knights Templar building and running hospitals for the Crusaders wherever they took their fight. With the advent of the military nursing orders, a harsher element entered nursing. There was an emphasis on rank and obedience to superior officers, although it is clear that there were huge strides forward during this period in the building of hospitals, the knights themselves nursing the patients (Austin 1957). Meighan (1990) claims that the early military roots of nursing have promoted controlling leadership styles in order to achieve greatest compliance with orders.

After the Crusades, organised care for the sick remained the province of religious and military orders if the family was unable to provide it, and nursing outside these institutions was informal and largely historically unrecorded. This religious and military background, with its connotations of altruism and obedience, still has an impact on modern nursing, but it was not until the 19th century that nursing in the UK received one of its most momentous shifts forward.

Florence Nightingale

It is not possible to discuss the history of nursing without mentioning Florence Nightingale, the woman who organised nursing for the first time in the UK in the latter half of the 19th century and who is probably the earliest British embodiment of a nursing 'leader' figure. From what we know of her through her biographers, she certainly wielded personal power and was able to influence the policy-makers of her time, but even she, strong as she was, allowed nursing to be dominated by the medical profession. It also seems clear that, although she had power and used it to great effect, she did not seem to be able to empower other nurses. It is this, I think, coupled with the dominance of medicine, that has had a lasting impact on the subsequent progress and development of nursing as a profession in its own right.

Miss Nightingale was a fine administrator, excellent at devising efficient systems and putting them into place, slicing her way through the red tape and bureaucracy of the day by using her social and family contacts. She was probably the first health service statistician, and reports and returns based upon her original format were adopted by a congress of London hospitals. This idea of collecting information was further developed by Sir Henry Burdett and was still being used by organisations such as the King Edward Hospital Fund as late as 1948 (Ives 1948).

The role of matron developed during this time as an autocratic figure, set apart from the rank and file of the working nurses. Indeed, Nightingale called her nurse managers 'Specials', and they were, like their counterpart leaders in the military, drawn from the higher social classes of the time and treated differently in terms of education and reward systems (Woodham-Smith 1950).

Reading a biography of Florence Nightingale, for example that by Woodham-Smith (1950), is highly recommended. Lytton Strachey (1948) wrote a fascinating account of her in his book *Eminent Victorians*. The section on Florence Nightingale from that book has been reproduced in collaboration with the Royal College of Nursing as a Penguin 60 edition. There is also an excellent two-volume biography by Sir E. T. Cook (1913), which, although out of print, is worth pursuing through libraries or second-hand book shops. In addition to these, there is a useful commentary in Margret Forster's book *Significant Sisters* (1989), which may be more accessible. Those whose knowledge of Florence Nightingale is based upon traditional views and notions of the 'lady with the lamp' will be surprised by what they read. She was an extremely tough woman who fought for years against her family to be allowed to become a nurse. Once trained, she manipulated friends and enemies alike to get her own way and pursue improvements for her patients. Florence Nightingale's methods are a study in political 'nous' and the very effective use of personality to influence others.

Carry On, Matron?

Fraser-Gamble, cited in Davidson and Cole (1991), claims that the autocratic matron led nursing services clearly and unambiguously until the 1960s. She also feels that the loss of the matron as the service head was a significant factor in nursing's later leadership problems. This view has occasionally been reiterated over the years, most significantly when the Griffiths Report of 1983 and the Audit Commission Report of 1991 expressed concerns over the perceived lack of management accountability in the service in general and referred sympathetically to the days when the matron would have known exactly what was happening in 'her' hospital and would have been firmly in charge – of everything.

There are, however, those who question this fond remembrance; Robinson, again cited in Davidson and Cole (1991), questioned the effectiveness of the matron figure in terms of any contribution to the advancement of practice and whether the exercising of such autocratic power had any lasting benefits. She claims that the matron was only able to exercise authority because she had support from the medical staff, and therefore her power was borrowed from the medical power base rather than arising out of genuine nursing knowledge and contribution. I personally wrote, in a heartfelt letter to the editor of *Nursing Times* (Girvin 1989), of negative personal experiences of matrons, again with the view that their power was autocratic and oppressive and did little to serve the needs of the profession in a developmental way. However, this type of 'command and control' approach does have its uses in some situations.

Discussion Points

Can you think of someone whom you would describe as autocratic?

What are the advantages of an autocratic style?

Can you think of a scenario in which a 'command and control' approach might be the best one to take?

Salmon: the 1960s and 70s

During the early 1960s, nursing was experiencing great difficulty in recruiting to the profession, and new approaches to retaining nurses in the service had to be considered. The outcome of the Salmon Report (1960) was to introduce an extensive nursing hierarchy in order to attract and retain staff by providing a clear upward career pathway, not dissimilar to the original principles behind the nursing clinical grading structure introduced in the late 1980s. This had a temporary effect on shortages because it was an attractive deal for nurses, but it created a much longer-term insidious problem by promoting unprepared clinical nurses into management positions. These new roles – nursing officers – were not always well thought through, and the post-holders often felt that their jobs had nothing to do with the introduction of new practices or the demonstration of clinical expertise. Consequently, many nursing officers became alienated from practice, reinforcing the already growing gap between management and practice (Jones *et al.* 1981).

Layers of hierarchy were introduced as a result of Salmon – nursing officers, senior nursing officers, principal nursing officers, chief nursing officers, divisional nursing officers and so on. Clinical nurses had, on the whole, little or no contact with the more senior levels and questioned their credibility from the start, although their rank and positional authority over nursing appeared to be maintained. It was at this time that nurse managers began to lose much of their power over related services such as housekeeping and domestic services.

Although the Salmon reforms ostensibly gave nurses the opportunity to influence strategic and policy-making levels, the success and influence within the service of these nursing officer roles has always been debated. My view is that this was usually more to do with the people in these posts, their skills and attributes, their interpretation of their role, than with the usefulness of the role itself. Sadly, this sort of confusion between personality and role function is still common in the service and can lead to the loss of crucial functions simply because a post-holder does not fulfil the role properly. The post gets scrapped as soon as there is an opportunity to do so, and what should have been useful functions disappear with it. Readers will undoubtedly be able to recognise occasions on which this has happened in their own organisations.

During the 1970s consensus management techniques were developing, which often meant more promotion for nurses; for example, nurses had a seat on health authorities and were expected to be involved in decision-making at that level. Ralph (cited in Jolley and Allen 1989) asserts that most were unfortunately simply not prepared for higher-level management practices and soon discovered that it was, in fact, quite difficult to influence colleagues during the decision-making process. In the culture of equality that was meant to underpin consensus management, many nurses were finding out that some of their colleagues seemed to be more equal than others. The assumptions that nurses had always held about the importance of their views were being challenged. From the late 1970s, the Salmon structures began to disintegrate. Over the next 10 years or so, the organisational structures of nursing went through numerous changes of role and title, but real power was rarely added (Savage 1990). Strong and Robinson (1988) have argued that, during this period, many nurses who possessed real leadership potential became very discouraged and either left the service or gave in to what appeared to be an oppressive and frustrating system. This meant that, as before, nursing was not well placed to take advantage of the radical changes that the 1980s would bring.

Discussion Points

Talk to someone who remembers the Salmon structures being in place. Do they remember them as positive or negative?

Salmon seemed at first to be successful. What do you think went wrong?

Discuss the notion of consensus management with your colleagues. What do you think led to its demise as an approach to managing health care?

Griffiths and Groping in the Dark

In the early 1980s, the government asked Roy Griffiths, best known at the time for his association with the food retailing giant Sainsbury's, to review the way in which the NHS was managed. The resulting NHS Management Enquiry of 1983 was critical of the unwieldy management structures, the lack of leadership and the procrastinating consensus management that had developed in the NHS. In simple terms, Griffiths' proposals included the introduction of simpler, flatter management structures, the devolvement of management responsibility to the lowest feasible level in the organisation, and a much more clearly defined upward accountability to general managers. Nursing functional hierarchies of management (in which nurses were managed by nurses) were stripped out at a stroke. The structures that Salmon had introduced to demonstrate the value and contribution that nurses ought to have throughout the service had succeeded only in demonstrating confusion, inaccessibility and a feeling of being out of touch with the reality of the business.

This was a huge blow to nurses' confidence, and, as a result of this and of being taken by surprise, nurses did not envisage themselves moving into the general manager roles promoted by Griffiths and did not apply for these positions in any numbers. The decentralisation process of the Griffiths reforms destroyed many of the existing ranks and roles in nursing. Because nurses had come to rely upon the security of functional management positions – that is, nurses managing nurses – they were ill equipped politically to compete against general managers for jobs. It quickly became clear that their voice in the new structures was much weaker, and they were in real danger of being completely marginalised.

Nurses were continuing to think in hierarchical terms after years of socialisation and tradition (Salvage 1990). Many senior nurses found themselves no longer required as managers and either returned to more practice-orientated functions or left the service for education or research. Nursing hierarchies had, at this time, been predominantly female, and as nurse manager roles disappeared, the NHS management culture created by the Griffiths reforms had an overwhelming male ethos (Clay 1986). The results of introducing general management seemed not only to be a step backward for nurses, but also to shift the balance against women. (Gender issues relating to leadership warrant more detailed discussion and will be addressed in Chapter 6.)

In January 1986 the Royal College of Nursing launched a campaign against general management reflecting the attack to their self-esteem that nurses felt they had suffered as a result of the Griffiths reforms. Nurses appeared to be demoralised and demotivated, and the cycle described by Burns (1978), of lack of motivation leading to lack of resources leading to lack of power, began to demonstrate itself. This negative cycle seems to be the dominant and even destructive ethos that pervaded nursing in the 1980s and early 1990s.

Discussion Points

How do you feel about line management structures for nurses? Discuss the advantages and disadvantages of being managed by someone from the same profession.

Why do you think nurses lost control of the nursing workforce?

Does it make a difference who manages nurses? Is this anyway a relevant debate in today's NHS?

It is not too difficult to see how these political and structural changes caused long-term problems for nurses. Even Kenneth Clarke, before he completed his term as Secretary of State for Health, recognised that removing functional management left unconnected and ambiguous strands of accountability (Davidson 1990). After the Griffiths reorganisations, when the impact of the lack of nurses at an influential level in the service began to be felt, it began to be more widely recognised that there was an urgent need to develop nurses for leadership positions in the NHS.

From the middle of the 1980s, nursing began to look seriously at the notion of leadership within the profession and its apparent lack. Although general management had offered new structures, giving nurses new opportunities to exercise leadership, this had felt to many like a leap in the dark. Preconceived ideas, of both managers and nurses, held many nurses back from seizing these opportunities (Kitching 1993). The introduction of Trust boards, requiring a nurse director to sit on the board, drew attention to the need for nurses to be prepared for executive level working and to the gaps in the career pathways and preparation processes that sometimes made these posts difficult to fill.

An attempt was made to try to increase the general profession's interest in the nature of and need for leadership in nursing by the publication of the Department of Health's *A Strategy for Nursing* (1989). This document contained a whole section on leadership and management, proposing seven action targets. The *Strategy* (p. 6) defined leadership as:

> setting the pace and direction for change, facilitating innovative practice, ensuring that policy is up to date, that professional standards are set in relation to care and that a comprehensive service is developed over time.

The *Strategy* came in for fierce criticism from some quarters. Salvage (1989) felt that the definition offered was simply a competency checklist and failed to take account of the more emotional factors of leadership. She also believed that the document did not recognise the difference between management and leadership. Salvage felt that nursing appeared to be unable to find effective leaders and that the Griffiths Report had highlighted this. Her views in the popular nursing press publicly reflected the disaffection between 'rank and file' nurses and their leaders that was so prevalent in the 1980s.

Discussion Points

Read *A Strategy for Nursing* (Department of Health, 1989) and discuss it with your colleagues.

Is it clear about leadership? Do you think it confuses management and leadership?

How might it have been improved so that it meant more to nurses?

Stopping the Rot

For many years, senior nurses had been exerting tight control over the mass of the workforce, largely by the power of their position. There had been few opportunities for nurses to develop leadership styles other than those related to the traditional power of position and rank, and 'command and control' styles, and the *Strategy* in many ways appeared to reinforce this. However, in spite of this criticism, the *Strategy* was a part of the process of nurses trying to explore the nature of leadership as it related to their own profession and of their beginning to be more constructive rather than simply bemoaning its lack.

American literature from around this period reveals a number of studies about nursing leadership that should have been considered. These describe how leadership style affects subordinate behaviour and how relationships are the key to effective leadership. For example, Nealey and Blood (1968) studied leadership style related to job satisfaction, and Pryor and Distefano (1971) reported on perceptions of leadership behaviour and job satisfaction. Both studies demonstrated a correlation between job satisfaction and considerate leadership behaviour. Duxbury *et al.* (1984) reported a similar correlation between considerate leadership style and staff burn-out. More recently, Pfaff (1987) and Longo and Uranker (1989) found that the most satisfying aspects of nurses' jobs were the positive relationships with their supervisors and co-workers.

A start was also being made on exploring and defining the qualities required by nurse leaders. Smith (1985) described these qualities as the ability:

- to think and be creative
- to show initiative and imagination
- to be courageous and have stamina.

He also reinforced the view of the importance of followers by remarking that nurses can only claim to be leaders when people are following them. Smith explored the fact that nurses are interdependent with the rest of the health care team and that old notions of autocracy and position power were unhelpful. He felt that nurse leaders of the future would need to be 'part pragmatist, part philosopher'.

Discussion Points

Discuss the statement 'part pragmatist, part philosopher'. What does it mean?

What combination of qualities and behaviours would you expect to see in someone who used this model?

Does this fit with your own ideas of what a nurse leader should be like? Why, or why not?

Throughout the nursing literature, a development in the understanding of the concept of leadership as applied to nursing is apparent in much the same way as is the development in more general leadership applications. This consists of a recognition of personality and style, and the development of specific skills, which mirrors the development from industry and commerce discussed in the early part of this book. As the need to understand leadership emerged, so reviews relating general leadership research to nursing appeared. Wilson (1980) clustered the leadership research literature into four themes:

- the personality of the leader
- the followers – their attitudes, needs and problems
- the groups – their characteristics
- the situation – the task.

This reflects the development already discussed that all of these factors must be taken into consideration as no single element can explain leadership in the nursing context. Chapter 5 opens our exploration of the development of leadership in nursing, through traditional approaches to the use of more contemporary ideas such as transformational leadership.

References

Audit Commission (1991) *The Virtue of Patients: Making Best Use of Ward Nursing Resources.* Audit Commission/HMSO. London.

Austin A (1957) *History of Nursing Source Book*. GP Putnams Sons. New York. Also cited in Donahue (1985).

Burns J (1978) *Leadership*. Harper & Row. New York.

Clay T (1986) Where have all the women gone? *Lampada*. Supplement.

Cook ET (1913) *The Life of Florence Nightingale*. Macmillan. London.

Davidson L (1990) Leading question. *Nursing Times*. 86(45): 16–17.

Davidson L and Cole A (1991) A crisis of leadership? *Nursing Times* 87(1): 22–5.

Department of Health, Nursing Division (1989) *A Strategy for Nursing*. Department of Health. London.

Donahue MP (1985) *Nursing – The Finest Art*. CV Mosby. Missouri.

Duxbury M, Armstrong G, Drew D and Henly S (1984) Head nurse leadership style with staff nurse burn-out and job satisfaction in neonatal intensive care units. *Nursing Research*. 33(2): 97–101.

Forster M (1989) *Significant Sisters: The Grass Roots of Active Feminism 1839–1939*. Penguin. London.

Girvin J (1989) Letter to the editor. *Nursing Times*. 85(8): 15.

Griffiths R (1983) *NHS Management Enquiry*. DHSS. London.

Ives A (1948) *British Hospitals*. Collins. London.

Jolley M and Allen P (eds) (1989) *Current Issues in Nursing*. Chapman & Hall. London.

Jones D, Crossley-Holland C and Matus I (1981) *The Role of the Nursing Officer*. DHSS. London.

Kitching D (1993) Nursing leadership – myth or reality? *Journal of Nursing Management*. 1: 253–7.

Longo R and Uranker M (1989) Why nurses stay: a positive approach to nursing shortage. *Nursing Management*. July: 78–9.

Meighan M (1990) The most important characteristics of nursing leaders. *Nursing Administration Quarterly*. 15(1): 63–9.

Nealey S and Blood M (1968) Leadership performance of nursing supervisors at two organisational levels. *Journal of Applied Psychology*. 52: 414–22.

Pfaff J (1987) Factors related to job satisfaction/dissatisfaction of registered nurses in long term facilities. *Nursing Management*. 18(8): 51–2.

Pryor M and Distefano M (1971) Perceptions of leadership behaviour, job satisfaction and internal/external locus of control across three nursing levels. *Nursing Research*. 20: 534–7.

Salmon B *et al.* (1966) *Report of the Committee on Senior Nursing Staff Structure*. The Salmon Report. HMSO. London.

Salvage J (1989) Take me to your leader. *Nursing Times*. 85(25): 34–5.

Savage P (1990) NHS reorganisations, leadership styles and nursing. *Senior Nurse*. 10(4): 6–8.

Smith J (1985) Qualities of leadership. *Nursing Mirror* **161**(11): 16–17.

Stewart IM (1918) How can we help to improve our teaching in nursing schools? *Canadian Nurse*. **22**: 1593. Also cited in Donahue (1985).

Stewart IM (1921) Popular fallacies about nursing education. *The Modern Hospital*. **18**(1) November. Also cited in Donahue (1985).

Strachey L (1948) *Eminent Victorians*. Penguin. London.

Strong P and Robinson J (1988) *New Model Management – Griffiths and the NHS*. University of Warwick. Coventry.

Wilson J (1980) A review of the literature and theoretical framework for nursing courses. *Nursing Leadership*. **3**(52): 32–8.

Woodham-Smith C (1950) *Florence Nightingale*. Constable. London.

The Royal College of Nursing has a forum for nurses interested in nursing history – The RCN History of Nursing Society. It publishes the *International History of Nursing Journal* three times a year. For further information contact RCN Headquarters at 20 Cavendish Square, London W1M OAB.

Chapter 5 The Story So Far...

This chapter contains a summary of the main features concerning the development of leadership theory in nursing and how it has mirrored the developments in more general fields, starting with exploring personal qualities and moving through to contingency approaches and choice. It also brings us up to date by taking a closer look at one of the latest and most popular developments in leadership theory so far – the concept of transformational leadership.

From our review of the nursing literature on leadership, we have seen that early work concentrates on qualities and personal traits: what sort of people should our leaders be? (Smith 1985; Salvage 1989; Davidson and Cole 1991). It goes on to take increasing account of the strategies that effective leaders use and to explore the notion of power related to leadership. In a particularly interesting commentary, Mackie (1987) describes leadership itself as a special form of power and claims that, whereas all leaders actually or potentially hold power, not all those who hold power are leaders. Mackie feels that, in nursing, we often confuse authority in the organisation with leadership, and this is a key factor in the apparent disappointment with those whom we see as our leaders. It can be agreed that this is a fundamental mistake in looking for leadership. We find it hard to identify leaders if they are not in traditional power positions, and, similarly, we expect those in traditional power positions to be leaders.

Mackie goes on to describe nurse leaders as working from two power bases: the power of resources and the power of motivation. Resources are defined as expertise, time, self-esteem, money and skill legitimacy, and Mackie explains that access to them or their deployment is used to influence the choices of others in the organisation. In addition, she feels that the underlying motivation of the nurse leader is crucial to the use of this resource power. This is an interesting thought; unfortunately, in searching through the literature, there appears to be little research specifically into the motivation of nurse leaders.

Mackie appears to have raised a good point here, particularly with her views on the confusion of authority with leadership: we look in the wrong places for leadership, expecting it to co-exist with managerial position and hierarchy, our expectations are misplaced and therefore thwarted, but there should be ways of avoiding this mismatch. This problem of misplaced expectation should inform the preparation and selection of both managers and leaders. In my view, all applicants for positions of authority in organisations should be required to demonstrate leadership skills, ability and achievement, or to commit themselves to a learning programme in order to develop those skills as a condition of appointment. It is small wonder that we continue to be disappointed if we expect leadership to occur naturally in people who are appointed to jobs only on the basis of their organisational management skills. As many of us can bear witness, good managers do not necessarily make good leaders.

Mackie's ideas on the two interrelated power bases are also interesting. I believe very strongly that motivation has a major part to play in effective leadership behaviour, and I have undertaken my own research into this (Girvin, forthcoming). Without digressing into too much detail, this study tried to examine the links between nurse executive directors' ability to carry out effective leadership behaviours and their motivation to stay in a particular job. The hypothesis was that motivation to stay in a leadership position within a particular organisation would correspond positively with the ability to demonstrate effective leadership behaviour. Early results indicate that motivation, job satisfaction and effective leadership in nurse executives are indeed linked. Motivation is discussed again in Chapter 7.

Discussion Points

Taking into account what you have read about nursing history, why do you think that some nurses might have been disappointed by their leaders?

Do you have aspirations to be a nurse leader, or are you already in a leadership position? If so, what made you want to be influential over your colleagues, what motivates you to lead?

Do you think that nurses are motivated by different things now than they were, for example, 20 or 50 years ago? If so, what are the differences? If not, why are the motivating factors of years ago still relevant?

Moving on from power and motivation, Baker (1983) clarified the importance of the group perspective in nursing leadership in her research into leadership at ward sister level. Baker's research described how the position power and authority of one ward sister was completely overturned by her subordinates. They were unimpressed by her performance, saw her actions as inept and unrealistic, and ultimately felt that they could do the job better themselves. The ward sister had failed to obtain any authority of knowledge and had, as a consequence, lost her authority of position. The perceptions of the group experiencing leadership are put succinctly by Armstrong (1988) when she talks about a leader being 'one of us, most of us, the best of us' and fitting into the followers' expectations of a leader for that situation. This demonstrates the enormous and sometimes overwhelming pressures on leaders to be all things to all people. They must be accepted as one of the group as well as being able to operate as guide, mentor and front person. This is a very tricky and fluid combination of roles to manage, requiring a battery of skills and significant personal insight.

Continuing with the theme of relationships between leaders and followers, group work approaches have been popularised in general nursing through the work of Alison Kitson and her colleagues in the 1980s and 90s in the Royal College of Nursing's Standards of Care and Dynamic Quality Improvement projects. Kitson promoted facilitated group work to bring about and lead improvements in the quality of care, and there is much anecdotal literature supporting the effectiveness of this approach (for example, Dunn 1990; Girvin 1991; Girvin and Baker 1991).

As part of an attempt to develop a higher profile in nursing leadership issues, the Royal College of Nursing produced a list of requirements, which, it was felt, would enhance nursing's ability to take on a stronger leadership role (MacPherson 1991). These factors, aimed at encouraging nurses to leave behind their traditional ideas of how leadership works, are:

- leading without relying on status or the position held
- having a vision for an organisation and the development of a framework to promote it
- inspiring confidence in others
- adaptability, facilitating easy movement from one leadership position to another.

MacPherson's list seems very well to reflect the environment in which nursing finds itself in the 1990s, an environment in which position power is very limited, in which personality (inspiration and motivation) must be used as a prime tool and in which career mobility is increasingly significant. All of these factors combine to produce a very responsive model of leadership, one that is eminently suitable for its time. Some of the factors on MacPherson's list will crop up later when we take stock of the fundamental aspects and attributes needed for effective leadership.

Discussion Points

Do you think that MacPherson's list reflects effective leadership behaviour?

What would you remove from it? Or add to it?

Is it a 'universal' list, appropriate for all levels of leadership?

Transformational Leadership

The concept of transformational leadership described by James MacDonald Burns has received a great deal of attention in the nursing press, both in the UK and in America, and shows no sign of losing its popularity. Burns (1978) has identified and compared two types of leadership: transformational and transactional.

Trofino (1993) offers a succinct paraphrasing of Burns' descriptions, explaining that transactional leadership occurs when leaders set up relationships with followers that are based on an exchange for some resource valued by the followers. Interactions between the transactional leader and the followers appear to be episodic, short-lived and limited to that one particular transaction.

In contrast to this, transformational leadership is much more complex and happens when people are engaged together in such a way that leaders and followers encourage one another to increased levels of motivation and morality. The aspirations of leaders and followers merge to become identical, and they develop a common purpose that can benefit the organisation, the profession and any other participants. Burns (1978) describes such leadership as being elevating, mobilising, inspiring, exalting, uplifting and evangelising. The key feature of transformational leadership is that it encourages followers to rise above their own goals and self-interests, and strive for the common good. It certainly sounds an attractive and appealing way of interacting with others.

There is a growing body of American literature describing the attributes and benefits of transformational leaders (Dunham and Klafehn 1990; McDaniel and Wolf 1992; Beecroft 1993). According to their way of thinking, nursing has, in the past, been largely transactional in its leadership processes, with a focus on the task and getting the job done. Transformational leadership, on the other hand, fits in with apparent desirable changes to our society and some work cultures in which there would be a focus less on task and more on job satisfaction and personal fulfilment.

Transformational leaders are able to articulate clearly their vision of the future. When they do this, they exhibit a style that is so attractive – inspiring and meaningful to others – that followers become strongly committed because the vision reflects and extends their own aspirations (Trofino 1995). Transformational leadership has also been described as being about change, innovation and entrepreneurship, encouraging the personal growth and empowerment of the leader and followers (Tichy and Devanna 1990). Zalesnik (1989) describes transformational leaders as those who arouse strong positive emotion and who can influence values, beliefs and behaviour. Bader and O'Malley (1992) assert that transformational leadership is about people, managing the corporate culture and having multiple strategies for change. They feel that transformational leaders have an innate ability to create vision in the hearts and minds of others, to seize opportunities and to empower staff at all levels. Bader and O'Malley (1992) also feel that such leaders have a 'magical ability to commit people to action'.

However, before we get too carried away by all this inspiration, shared vision and commitment, what does all this really mean – in practical terms? This concept of leadership seems to embrace management effectiveness coupled with charisma and an accurate assessment of the values and higher-level motivators of the workforce: it describes someone who can put into words what the majority of people hope for the future, someone who can express those aspirations in terms of a series of specific actions and objectives and then something a little less tangible, someone who can make others feel that it is possible to do things that they have until now only dreamed of. It is a clever combination of personal qualities and specific functions and actions that has caught everyone's imagination, a heady mixture of rhetoric and reality that can make the ultimate difference.

Tichy and Devanna (1990) feel that it is a very deliberate set of actions, a systematic process of searching for changes, and that its prime activities are behavioural processes that can be learned. Transformational leadership has also been described as having additional 'spin-off' benefits, such as enhancing staff retention and satisfaction (Dunham and Klafehn 1990; McDaniel and Wolf 1992).

Dunham and Klafehn (1990), writing specifically about nurse leaders, undertook a study of those leaders identified by their peers and subordinates as being 'excellent' and determined which of the skills they employed were associated with a transformational leadership style. The skills and qualities associated with transformational leadership style were considered to be:

- decision-making ability
- commitment
- demonstrating a long-term vision of what can be accomplished and identifying common values with staff
- having the ability to inspire others with that vision and to empower others to do the best they can within the shared value system.

The authors compared the results of those demonstrating transformational traits with others who demonstrated transactional traits. They concluded from this that transactional leaders acted only in a 'caretaker' capacity, with no vision for the future and no overtly shared values. Any changes implemented by transactional leaders were deemed to be 'first order' changes – changes of process or procedure rather than system or cultural change. In comparison, they felt that transformational leaders made 'second order' changes – changes that would have a lasting benefit because they changed systems and views and ways of thinking. Dunham and Klafehn (1990) went on to describe three stages of development from transactional towards transformational leadership behaviour:

- transactional stage 1: The leader's personal goals and agendas take precedence
- transactional stage 2: The leader's personal needs are achieved; he or she understands and participates in mutual experiences and shared partnerships
- transformational stage 3: The leader develops end values and considers them to be more important than the group agenda and loyalties. The leader's decisions are based on those end values rather than on allegiance to the group.

This study demonstrated that those nurse executives who were perceived to be excellent had transformational skills and qualities (and that those skills were recognised and valued by their staff). It also suggested that choice is crucial – choice of when to use the transformational techniques of charisma, consideration and intellectual stimulation, and when to use the transactional techniques of contingent reward and management by exception. Earlier, we explored the notion of charisma and discussed its use as a leadership tool rather than as an inherent personal quality. This will be revisited only briefly here.

Davidhizar (1993) sees charisma as an important characteristic that can be useful for leaders who want to motivate by interpersonal means rather than authoritarian approaches. According to Davidhizar, utilising charisma in leadership involves a number of elements, including:

- communicating positive self-esteem
- focusing on people
- having a vision
- promoting the vision
- implementing the vision.

It is useful to draw attention to these descriptors of charisma because they are very closely linked to the features of transformational leadership.

As in everything, there is a balance to be sought between transformational and transactional leadership, and elements of both of these types of leadership probably need to be present in the same individual in order to be able to respond to the greatest variety of situations and still have consistent success.

Further research by Bass *et al.* (1987), cited in Dunham and Klafehn (1990), supports this by suggesting that transformational leadership may not be as effective when used on its own; the authors believe that it may well act as an enhancer and supporter of transactional interventions. This reinforces the point made in the earlier chapters of this book about good leaders having a choice of styles and interventions available to them, so that they can decide upon and implement the most effective response for the specific situation.

Discussion Points

What do you think are the differences between transformational and transactional leadership?

Can you recognise these two styles in any leaders whom you know?

Discussion Points *(cont'd)*

Think of a few charismatic leaders. What is it that makes them charismatic?

Do you think that it is possible to learn this skill, or do you have to be born with it?

Is acting part of the leadership skills portfolio? (This is a serious question.)

Another recent theory of leadership associated with nursing appears to be that of 'connective leadership' (Klakovich 1994). Klakovich maintains that Burns' (1978) original notion of transformational leadership has an emphasis on competition and conflict, and she suggests a more affiliative paradigm, called connective leadership, which is based on work by Lipman-Blumen. Lipman-Blumen (1994, cited by Klakovich 1994), defines connective leadership as collaborative, contributory, mentoring, interactive in style, trusting, empowering, networking and persuasive. Differentiation between these two theories is not, on the basis of the present review of the literature, very clear. What it does seem to do is gather together all the most positive aspects of personality, style, behaviour and contingent approaches to leadership and call it connective leadership. Whether it is actually a new theory is debatable.

There is a new paradigm of leadership emerging: the post-industrial paradigm proposed by Rost (1994), which appears to be a significant new conception of leadership. Rost rejects what he calls the industrial paradigm of leadership as 'good management' and proposes that leadership is a relationship that is defined by four essential elements:

1. Both leaders and collaborators are involved in the relationship
2. They use only non-coercive influence strategies in that relationship
3. They intend significant changes
4. They make sure that the changes reflect the mutual purposes of both the collaborators and the leaders.

Rost (1994) uses the term 'collaborator' instead of 'follower' in order to convey the sense of involvement that there must be in a leadership relationship as opposed to the connotations of a passive carrying out of instructions, which the term 'follower' implies. Rost's exciting new approach considers leadership to be something positive, mutually respectful and concerned with leading and living in times of transformational change. He rejects the idea that leadership cannot be defined or is even difficult to define. He sees leadership as a process, an episodic process that happens from time to time rather than continuously. Rost's is a refreshing, straight-between-the-eyes view of leadership. Reading Rost's article (1994) and book (1991), details of which can be found at the end of the chapter, will stimulate ideas of how nursing leadership needs to develop.

Having considered the history and politics of nursing leadership thus far, and also briefly touched on what appear to be the latest leadership theories, we should turn our attention to what is happening to nursing leadership in the face of all these changes and developments. What are we learning, as a profession, and how are we making the most of new developments in leadership approaches?

It would appear that, in the UK, the NHS and the Department of Health are showing a growing understanding of the need to separate management and leadership as concepts and are trying to promote a consistent approach to the nurturing of leadership skills through the document *A Vision for the Future* (Department of Health/NHSE 1993). This document contains targets meant to help the profession to encourage and develop leadership skills in addition to recognising and developing potential leaders throughout the organisation. The 'Vision' document avoids the pitfalls into which the earlier *Strategy for Nursing* (1989) fell by clearly recognising the need for leadership at all levels of the organisation – in clinical practice, in management, in education, in policy-making and in politics. There has also been an effort to follow these targets through by asking organisations to demonstrate their action through an informal monitoring process, which resulted in the report *Testing the Vision* (Department of Health/NHSE 1994). Results appear impressive in this document, but there is not much detail and it still falls back into talking about management and leadership in the same breath.

Leadership training is becoming more widespread. The King's Fund runs courses for nurses and others at different stages of leadership development and for different levels in the organisation. The Royal College of Nursing's leadership project is gaining momentum, and it has produced a range of literature to help nurses decide where on the continuum of leadership development they might be and what actions to take next.

It would thus appear that nursing seems to be gaining a better understanding of leadership and the skills required to develop successful leaders. It still needs to find better ways of communicating, which will help to bridge the gap between those perceived as leaders and those looking for or needing leadership, and help organisations to realise that a position of authority in the organisation does not automatically confer leadership.

However, in spite of these steps forward, we still, according to the views of the rank and file of nurses represented in the popular nursing press, seem to lack leaders. Nursing's history and its politics are only a part of this story – there are a number of other important influences that must be considered. Chapter 6 will look at how traditional attitudes and socialisation have affected nursing and the development of leadership.

Discussion Points

What are your personal views of nurse leaders, both national and more local ones?

What has influenced your views?

What would you be doing differently if you were in their position?

Do you think that nursing lacks leaders? If so, why? If not, why are they not better recognised?

What does the organisation in which you work do to encourage leaders and their development?

References

Armstrong M (1988) *A Handbook of Human Resources Management.* Kogan Page. London.

Bader G and O'Malley J (1992) Transformational leadership in action: an interview with a health care executive. *Nursing Administration Quarterly.* **17**(1): 38–44.

Baker D (1983) Care in the geriatric ward – an account of two styles of nursing. In Wilson-Barnett J (ed.) *Nursing Research.* John Wiley. Chichester.

Bass BM, Avolio BJ and Goodheim L (1987) Biography and the assessment of transformational leadership at world class level. *Journal of Management.* Jan. 7–19. Also cited in Dunham and Klafehn (1990).

Beecroft M (1993) Where are the transformational leaders? *Clinical Nurse Specialist.* **7**(4): 163.

Burns J (1978) *Leadership.* Harper & Row. New York.

Davidhizar A (1993) Leading with charisma. *Journal of Advanced Nursing.* **18**: 675–9.

Davidson L and Cole A (1991) A crisis of leadership? *Nursing Times.* **87**(1): 22–5.

Department of Health, Nursing Division (1989) *A Strategy for Nursing.* DoH. London.

Department of Health and National Health Service Executive (1993) *A Vision for the Future – the Nursing, Midwifery and Health Visiting Contribution to Health and Health Care.* DoH. London.

Department of Health and National Health Service Executive (1994) *Testing the Vision – a Report on Progress in the First Year of 'A Vision for the Future'.* DoH. London.

Dunham J and Klafehn K (1990) Transformational leadership and the nurse executive. *Journal of Nursing Administration.* **20**(4): 28–33.

Dunn C (1990) Improving intensive care. *Nursing Times.* **85**(41): 34–6.

Girvin J (1991) Deals on meals. *Nursing Times.* **87**(34): 38–40.

Girvin J (forthcoming) *Motivation and Satisfaction Factors Relating to Nurse Executive Directors.* Royal College of Nursing. London.

Girvin J and Baker C (1991) Standard setting in paediatrics. *Nursing Standard.* **5**(25): 32–4.

Klakovich M (1994) Connective leadership for the 21st century: a historical perspective and future directions. *Advanced Nursing Science.* **16**(4): 42–54.

McDaniel C and Wolf G (1992) Transformational leadership in nursing service. *Journal of Nursing Administration.* **22**(2): 60–5.

Mackie L (1987) The leadership challenge. *Senior Nurse.* **6**(4): 23.

MacPherson W (1991) Leadership is about change. *Nursing Standard.* **5**(36): 51.

Rost JC (1994) Leadership: a new conception. *Holistic Nursing Practice.* **9**(1): 1–8.

Salvage J (1989) Take me to your leader. *Nursing Times.* **85**(25): 34–5.

Smith J (1985) Qualities of leadership. *Nursing Mirror.* **161**(11): 16–17.

Tichy NM and Devanna MA (1990) *The Transformational Leader.* John Wiley. New York.

Trofino J (1993) Transformational leadership: the catalyst for successful change. *International Nursing Review.* **40**(6): 179–82, 187.

Trofino J (1995) Transformational leadership in health care. *Nursing Management.* **26**(8): 42–7.

Zalesnik A (1989) *The Management Mystique – Restoring Leadership in Business.* Harper & Row. London.

Further Reading

RCN Nurses in Leadership Project (1995) *A Guide to Planning Your Career.* Royal College of Nursing. London.

RCN Nurses in Leadership Project (1996) *Developing Leaders – a Guide to Good Practice.* Royal College of Nursing. London.

Rost JC (1991) *Leadership for the Twenty First Century.* Praeger. New York.

Chapter 6 Traditional Attitudes and Socialisation

In previous chapters, I have tried to clarify how nursing's apparent failure to produce effective leaders in sufficient quantities is a product of its social and political history. Hempstead (1992) claims that nurses are prisoners of their own past – steeped in tradition, comfortable in hierarchical structures and comfortable with management in a conventional, controlled environment. In the past, matrons exercised their power through their medical colleagues, consensus management in the 1970s meant that risk-taking was uncommon, and layers of functional management tiers meant that responsibility could be avoided relatively easily. Because of the profession's dependence upon functional structures (nurses managing nurses), leading to the confusion of management of the service with leadership (MacPherson 1991), nurses were simply not demonstrating the right skills or attitudes to make an impact after the implementation of the Griffiths recommendations in the 1980s.

Robinson and Strong (1987) and Strong and Robinson (1988) began to draw attention to the disastrous effect that this was having upon nursing. They reported that many nurses left the service in the mid to late 1980s because they simply could not face the dismissive attitudes and marginalisation that general management often brought. In addition to this, traditional nursing education and years of socialisation into the service made it difficult for them to accept accountability to anyone other than another professional. The gulf between nurses and managers was rapidly widening and would set a pattern of hostility for the future that is both negative and harmful. Clinical nurses, who had felt alienated from their own nurse managers since the Salmon structure reforms in the 1960s, were largely unsympathetic. In fact, many may have been pleased to see layers of perceived ineffectual nurse managers disappear. They saw it as an opportunity to get these people off their backs. Titles and positions had provided a veneer of leadership to people who really possessed few of the necessary skills once they were forced out from behind the cover of their positional authority (Hunt 1992).

Equally frustrating was the apparent naiveté concerning the input that was required to address these problems and to develop new kinds of leader for the future. Robinson, quoted in Davidson and Cole (1991), says with exasperation, 'a number of nurses are spotted as potential leaders at ward level, but people don't seem to realise the investment that has to be made in such a promotion – both in terms of education and in the preparedness to stand up and be counted. My hunch is that the best either have to capitulate to the status quo or find they are so unpopular with colleagues they have to get out.' This sums up very well what remains a persistent tension in nursing – that of bemoaning the lack of leadership while denigrating or disparaging those who are trying to provide it because their actions often challenge existing ways of thinking and working. Without the support of their own kind, from subordinates and peers, nurses had little chance of enlisting support from general managers.

By 1991 the principle of general management was well established, and there were few general managers with a nursing background (Davidson and Cole 1991). This has improved considerably at middle management levels as organisations have realised the benefits of having someone in charge who knows the business inside out, but numbers appear to remain small at the most senior levels of organisations. For example, information on the exact number of chief executives in England with a nursing qualification proved to be elusive.

In the early 1990s, nursing felt increasingly powerless and was becoming internally divided and therefore less able to give the kind of broad-based, positive support that emerging, stronger leaders needed (Hempstead 1992). A vicious circle seemed to be appearing: unless it could provide strong leaders, nursing would remain powerless and divided; as long as it felt powerless and divided it was unable to support strong leaders.

Changing demography and social expectations were probably also having an impact. There were more employment opportunities for women as part-time working increased and the recessions of the 1980s encouraged the entry of cheaper labour of women into the market. More and more women felt that it was socially unnecessary and undesirable to dedicate a life to nursing. Outside commitments began to take precedence, and nursing was unfortunately late to recognise that a career did not necessarily mean a full-time, childless, partnerless commitment to the profession. Offering flexible working patterns to nurses who wanted to return to work after a break to have a family or care for dependants was almost unheard of, and even now, in times of particular staff shortage, Trusts with really creative and flexible recruitment and retention policies are the exception rather than the rule (Audit Commission 1997).

Discussion Points

Why did nurses fail to develop their influence during the health service reforms of the early 1990s?

Do you think that this had an impact on the service?

Do you see nursing behaving in a different way as a result of these experiences?

Wright, cited in Davidson and Cole (1991), felt that the search for nursing leaders was too narrowly focused. He felt that nursing was continuing to fail to understand that leadership could exist at other than top levels of management, again noting the persistent confusion between leadership and management that seems still not to be addressed. On the other hand, clinical nurses did not value their 'managerial' colleagues and therefore did not value the people they perceived as their leaders at a time when it was crucial to reintroduce a nursing perspective to the management of the service. Wright believed that there were many more ways in which nurses could use power and influence other than through line management, but nurses have been slow to recognise the alternative power sources of knowledge and charisma, and translate them into ways of influencing organisations.

It took almost the complete removal of nurses from influential positions before the profession at large began to realise that it needed to take some action. The acceptance of the need for nurse leaders is a relatively recent development, not only among other professional groups and general managers, but also among some sections of the profession itself. Historically, as we have seen, the culture of nursing has not encouraged the development of leaders, largely because the traditionally accepted role of nurses has been to follow (Hunt 1992). If nursing is truly to get back into the picture of being influential in the service, it must become a much more unified profession, measuring leaders by their achievements and effectiveness. It is sad to see colleagues dismiss people who could give them considerable help simply because they are no longer engaged in practice. Nurses who are actively engaged in practice will always have difficulty in finding time to participate in the kind of long-drawn-out activities that form part of decision-making in organisations. Instead, they must find leaders who will reflect their point of view, who will tap their expertise when making a case for resources but who are able to spend time on the arguing, lobbying and preparation. They must use their leaders to make sure that the clinical viewpoint is a strong one. This cannot happen if clinical and non-clinical nurses do not respect, support and actively utilise each other.

This kind of in-fighting has held the profession back for years and been an easy weapon for others to exploit in their favour.

Discussion Points

Is there a framework within your organisation for clinical nurses to discuss issues and present their thoughts to local leaders of the profession, nurse executives for example?

If there is not, what can you do to remedy this?

What do you do to support your local nurse leaders at work and help them to do their job?

Are there ways in which these relationships could be improved?

Woman's Work

The lack of success that nurses experienced in obtaining influential positions may have been influenced by their gender. Nursing remains predominantly a female profession, and women have been aspiring to leadership positions for some time, with limited success (Agonito 1993). There is still a view that women do not make such effective leaders as men, and certain leadership behaviours have indeed been associated with the gender of leaders. Females have been reported to be more considerate in their approach compared with males, who take a more initiating approach (Makin *et al.* 1989). Often, if workers are used to a man as leader taking a particular approach, women suffer from the response described by Terborg (1977), that is, failing to adopt the expected leadership approach affects the satisfaction of subordinates and leads to a perception of the leader as 'bad' rather than 'different'. This is an appealingly easy answer to some of the difficulties experienced by women in positions of leadership. Just to show that there are no easy answers, however, Petty and Brunning (1980), in a large-scale study of men and women, failed to confirm this hypothesis. Nevertheless, there does seem to be a deeply entrenched view in our society that women do not make such good leaders as men. Agonito (1993) is quite clear that women who are perceived as powerful are rarely able to maintain an image as a 'nice girl'. Power and women is an uncomfortable combination for many people in the workplace.

Austin *et al.* (1985) undertook a study of how the words 'nurse' and 'feminine' were perceived in 30 language/culture communities. They found that the interpretation of the word 'nurse' occurred in a very similar way to the interpretation of the word 'feminine'. It was perceived as meaning 'good' and 'active' but also 'emotional' and 'weak'. This puts another potential barrier in front of nurses, who want to be judged on their actual abilities rather than on assumptions based on their gender. It seems that to be a powerful nurse can be bad enough, but to be a powerful nurse *and* a woman is a 'double whammy' that appears to be just too much for some die-hards to take.

There is also a view that women are fearful of being successful and therefore underestimate their abilities and are unwilling to put themselves forward for promotion (Davidson and Cooper

1992). Back in the 1970s Horner (1970) suggested that appearing to be successful was not behaving in a socially approved manner for a woman, and therefore, unwilling to face disapproval, women did not place themselves for promotion. This may have been a reasonable assumption 30 years ago, but it is a much less valid explanation in the post-feminist environment of today. Marshall (1984) suggests that it is fear of demonstrating an inappropriate gender role, rather than fear of social disapproval, that holds women back and that this is a response common to both men and women. Bordwick (1979) had already shown that men experience fears similar to women's when they undertake occupational roles not usually associated with their gender. This association of role and gender also affects the way in which subordinates respond. If subordinates feel that the 'leader' has an inappropriate gender role – a woman in a man's job or vice versa – their perception of that leader's performance is affected by these views (Peterson 1985).

Isolation and the lack of female role models may also be a factor in holding women back from leadership positions (Davidson and Cooper 1983; Marshall 1984; Asplund 1988; Powell 1988). This may have particular connotations for nursing, where women in very senior positions, executive nurses for example, may often be lone women in an all-male team. Where women join a well-established all-male team, acceptance on equal terms can be particularly difficult. If there are no local precedents, and if the team is not particularly sophisticated in its operation, this can be a nightmare scenario for many women as they struggle to be equal partners. Organisational culture is extremely important in situations like this as the signals given out by team members, no matter how slight, can make or break the future effectiveness of the newcomer. Yet organisations that have operated in a sexist manner – whether intentionally or subconsciously – need to have senior women role models in order to reassure their workforce, particularly where that workforce is predominantly women, as in nursing. This means that serious female role models are accepted and treated as equals, not just token women on the board or in the senior management team. Informal signals can be very powerful in setting the scene for the whole organisation.

Numerous studies show that female role models in higher leadership positions act as important influences in terms of career aspirations for other women (Davidson 1985; Freeman 1990). If we return specifically to nursing, it seems likely that nurses looking to senior positions following Griffiths, with its development of a male ethos, found very few female role models in those early years.

The history of female roles and female expectations, coupled with historical nursing roles and nursing socialisation, appear to be very powerful factors when considering the development of nursing and nursing leadership.

What Do We Need To Do?

It is essential that nurses understand how important effective leadership is if they are to be influential enough to secure patient welfare and to progress the aims of the profession in supporting health care systems. It appears that there are many nurses now in senior positions who do understand this need and have recognised that preparation for leadership roles is vital and must start at an early stage (Department of Health/NHSE 1993). This recognition is being turned into specific actions, and a concerted effort is being made by a number of organisations.

On the other hand, it has also been observed that the traditional networks of senior nurses have not been as effective at promoting the interests of their members as have many other professional groups (Lorentzon 1992). It has long been suspected, if not openly acknowledged, that where other professional groups are supportive and close knit in times of adversity, nurses can often be found being divisive and distancing themselves. Tales of the nursing network being 'unkind' to colleagues are not hard to find. National nursing networks need to take greater account of this and work hard to make it unnacceptable. Ignoring these more unpleasant aspects of the profession will not make them go away. Instead, it encourages people to think that they can get away with denigrating and disparaging; all it does is feed the notion that we do not have decent leaders, that we are being sold down the river and that we are a powerless and introspective profession. It is unattractive and turns us into victims of our own feelings of helplessness.

Nurse leaders, meaning all nurse leaders rather than those traditionally in the public eye, have to become much more visible and accessible if public perception of their importance – the relevance and validity of their opinion – is to change. We do not often *see* the opinion of nurses being sought in general health debates. For example, compare how many times a spokesperson for the medical profession appears on television compared with one for nursing. It seems that when the media require a clinical viewpoint, it is the medical opinion that is sought. This may seem trivial, but it represents an important issue.

Discussion Points

Consider your own organisation: what is the ratio of men to women in your senior management team?

How many women are there on your Trust board?

Ask your human resources department for the Trust's equal opportunities policy. Are there specific policies on harassment and gender discrimination?

If you can, invite someone who has been the subject of sexist behaviour at work to talk to a group. Try to get a female and a male perspective. Men in nursing are a minority group and frequently feel discriminated against. Sexism is sexism – it is irrelevant which gender it is directed against.

What Are We Doing To Encourage Leaders?

As mentioned above, there a number of initiatives already taking place with the purpose of fostering leaders for the future and further developing today's leaders. Most of this is aimed at more senior levels of the profession, but there is a growing recognition of the need to start identifying leadership potential early and to encourage leadership skills.

The need for an executive nurse network was identified in the late 1980s through the King's Fund Centre in London. This organisation later developed a number of very specific training courses for nurse executives to help them to develop what was then a new role. In 1991 the King's Fund developed learning sets for future nurse leaders, which have been a particularly successful way of bringing people together to debate similar problems and talk about their successes and failures in a non-threatening, non-competitive environment. There are also mentorship schemes arising from these initiatives, in which experienced nurse executives take a particular interest in someone who is expecting to develop as a nurse leader. Mentorship is a key activity in leadership and will be discussed in Chapter 8.

In 1992 Opportunity 2000 was established by the government as an initiative designed to increase the number of women holding managerial positions in all areas of employment. As a direct result of this, the NHS Women's Unit was set up with the specific purpose of helping more women into management positions within the NHS. The Women's Unit ran a successful network and offered training and personal coaching for women who needed encouragement and practical help to pursue a high-level career. It also administered a bursary scheme, which supported women undertaking higher education in related subjects, for example Masters degrees in Business Administration and other health-related subjects. This work has developed and enlarged its scope to cover a wider range of career aspirants and provides assistance for both men and women at middle management level. Changes in administration mean that it is now largely run by the Institute of Health and Care Development, based in Bristol.

Help for senior managers is currently provided by 'Executive Choice', a programme run by Dearden Management with the Health Service Management Unit in Manchester.

There are a number of additional networks for nurse executives – the Trust Nurses Association, the RCN's Executive Nurse Forum, and less formally many regions offer opportunities for nurse executives to get together. In addition, many nurse executives maintain their own personal networks of friends and colleagues.

Some regions have developed 'fast-tracking' systems that identify potential leaders early through a battery of managerial and personality tests and then push them through development training, depending upon their aptitude (Carlisle 1991).

75

Lower down in the organisation, it seems still to be very much up to individual employers to provide leadership development. Networking is most often found through specialist fora such as the Royal College of Nursing's special interest groups or through union branch meetings and conferences. As mentioned above, the RCN also has a leadership project aimed specifially at clinical nurses.

We are still not doing enough to nurture leadership skills before nurses find themselves in jobs that rely upon a whole range of skills that are relatively new to them. The next section of this book will attempt to define what those skills and requirements are and how we can make sure that learning about them is accessible to a greater number of nurses, from a much earlier stage in their career.

There may well be other initiatives that have been developed in the time up to the publication of this book. Up-to-date information can be found through professional journals, the local university library, the National Boards and professional organisations.

References

Agonito R (1993) *No More Nice Girl – Power, Sexuality and Success in the Work place*. Bob Adams. Massachusetts.

Asplund G (1988) *Women Managers – Changing Organisational Cultures*. John Wiley. Chichester.

Audit Commission (1997) *Finders, Keepers – The Management of Staff Turnover in NHS Trusts*. Audit Commission. London.

Austin J, Champion V and Tzeng O (1985) Cross-cultural comparison on nursing image. *International Journal of Nursing Studies*. 22 March: 231–9.

Bordwick J (1979) *In Transition*. Rhinehart & Winston. London.

Carlisle D (1991) On a fast track to the top. *Nursing Times*. **86**(51): 18.

Davidson M (1985) *Reach for the Top – a Woman's Guide to Success in Business and Management*. Piatkus. London.

Davidson L and Cole A (1991) A crisis of leadership? *Nursing Times*. **87**(1): 25.

Davidson M and Cooper C (1983) *Stress and the Woman Manager*. Martin Robertson. London.

Davidson M and Cooper C (1992) *Shattering the Glass Ceiling – the Woman Manager*. PCP. London.

Department of Health and National Health Service Executive (1993) *A Vision for the Future – the Nursing, Midwifery and Health Visiting Contribution to Health and Health Care*. DoH. London.

Freeman SJ (1990) *Managing Lives – Corporate Women and Social Change*. University of Massachusetts Press. Amherst. Cited in Davidson M and Cooper C (1992) *Shattering the Glass Ceiling – the Woman Manager*. PCP. London.

Hempstead N (1992) Nurse management and leadership today. *Nursing Standard*. **6**(33): 37–9.

Horner H (1970) *Femininity and Successful Achievement: A Basic Inconsistency. Feminine Personality and Conflicts*. Brookes Cole. California. Cited in Davidson M and Cooper C (1992) *Shattering the Glass Ceiling – the Woman Manager*. PCP. London.

Hunt J (1992) Nursing leadership opportunities. *Senior Nurse*. **12**(1): 13–15.

Lorentzon M (1992) Authority, leadership and management in nursing (guest editorial). *Journal of Advanced Nursing*. **17**: 525–7.

MacPherson W (1991) Leadership is about change. *Nursing Standard*. **5**(36): 51.

Makin P, Cooper C and Cox C (1989) *Managing People at Work*. British Psychological Society. Leicester.

Marshall J (1984) *Women Managers – Travellers in a Male World*. John Wiley. Chichester.

Peterson MF (1985) Experienced acceptability: measuring perception of dysfunctional leadership. *Group and Organisational Studies*. **10**: 447–77.

Petty M and Brunning N (1980) A comparison of the relationships between subordinates behaviour and measures of subordinates job satisfaction for them and for their leaders. *Academy of Management Journal*. **23**(4): 717–25. Cited in Davidson M and Cooper C (1992) *Shattering the Glass Ceiling – the Woman Manager*. PCP. London.

Powell G (1988) *Women and Men in Management*. Sage. London.

Robinson J and Strong P (1987) *Professional Nursing Advice after Griffiths – an Interim Report*. Warwick Nursing Policy Studies Centre. Warwick.

Strong P and Robinson J (1988) *New Model Management – Griffiths and the NHS*. University of Warwick. Coventry.

Terborg J (1977) Working women and stress. In Beehr T and Bhagat R (eds) *Human Stress and Cognition in Organisations*. John Wiley. Chichester.

Additional Information

The Institute of Health and Care Development, St Bartholomews Court, 18 Christmas Street, Bristol BS1 5BT.

RCN Nurses in Leadership Project, RCN HQ, 20 Cavendish Square, London W1M 0AB.

'Executive Choice', Dearden Management, Church Road, Redhill, Bristol BS18 7SG.

Chapter 7 Motivation

In the previous chapters, we touched briefly on motivation as it is related to leadership. This chapter will explore some of the most commonly cited literature on motivation and attempt to describe the development of motivation theory. Although motivation is considered in the general and nursing research literature to be crucial to the way in which leaders apply their skills and influence (McClelland 1975; Burns 1978; Mackie 1987), there is little research in nursing to demonstrate the motivations of effective nurse leaders. The literature on nurse leadership that touches on motivation appears to accept and assume the same motivation factors for nurse leaders as for other leaders. However, this could be an erroneous assumption as some research suggests that there are significant differences in motivation factors in terms of preferred rewards between professional leaders and other types of leader (Miner 1982). It appears that there may also be a gender factor to be considered – both Albarn-Metcalfe (1989) and Nicholson and West (1988) have found differences between the sexes in ambition and motivating factors.

The motivation to *be* a leader has been clearly researched in the general field and applied to nursing. The motivation to *stay* a leader is, however, much less clear. As we discussed earlier in the book, some of today's nurse leaders have defied history, politics and socialisation to obtain the positions they now occupy (Savage 1990; Kitching 1993). Some of them have had to deal on a daily basis with open hostility, sexism and dismissive attitudes once in more senior positions. In the face of such adversity – both in becoming and then operating as a leader – the motivators, if they can be identified, ought to be of enormous help in selecting and preparing future leaders.

Motivation is a term used to describe the entire collection of drives, desires, needs, wishes and similar forces that affect our will to do certain things. To be motivated is to carry out certain activities in the hope that these drives and desires will be satisfied by the action taken and the outcome of those actions (Koontz and Weihrich 1988).

It is widely accepted that human motives are based on conscious and unconscious needs, and that these needs can be divided into the two following broad categories:

1. primary needs – including purely physical requirements for water, air, food, sleep and shelter
2. secondary needs – including self-esteem, status, affiliation with others, affection, giving, accomplishment and self-assertion.

The concept of motivation has itself been described as a kind of chain reaction. It starts with the experience of needs, these needs then giving rise to specific wants or the identification of goals. Once the needs and related goals are identified, this gives rise to tension (or unfulfilled desires), which in its turn drives action towards achieving the goals, satisfying the wants and relieving the needs.

Maslow and Herzberg

One of the most widely known theories of motivation is the 'hierarchy of needs' theory put forward by Maslow (1954). Maslow placed a number of human needs into an ascending hierarchy. He took the view that until each layer of need was sufficiently satisfied, other needs would not become motivating factors. His layers of need began with the physiological, moving through security and safety, affiliation and acceptance, and then esteem until the highest order need was reached – that of self-actualisation.

Although popular for some years, Maslow's hierarchy has come increasingly under question. Lawler and Suttle (1972), in a study of 187 managers, found very little evidence to support the theory that human needs form a multistepped, ascending hierarchy. They did, however, note that there were two levels of need – 'biological' and 'other' – and that the 'other' only emerged when the biological needs had been satisfied. They also found that, at the higher level of 'other' needs, the strength of those needs varied from individual to individual. Thus, once basic needs are met, the motivation to satisfy the higher-order needs may or may not follow, depending upon the individual. Hall and Nougaim (1968), on the other hand, studied managers over a 5-year period and found no strong evidence of a needs hierarchy. They did, however, find that as managers became successful and were promoted upwards, their physiological and safety needs became less important and their need for affiliation, esteem and self-actualisation increased. However, the authors believed that this was due to the social implications of upward career changes and not a result of the satisfaction of lower-order needs.

Herzberg *et al.* (1957, 1959) modified Maslow's work considerably. Like Hall and Nougaim, they claimed a 'two-factor' theory of motivation. One factor group included policy and administration, supervision, working conditions, interpersonal relationships, salary, status and personal life. Herzberg *et al.* claim that these were dissatisfiers rather than motivators. In simple terms, they believed that if these elements existed in sufficient quality and quantity, people would, broadly speaking, be satisfied in their work – these factors would cause no dissatisfaction. They did not in themselves motivate, but their lack would result in dissatisfaction. Herzberg *et al.* called these 'hygiene' factors. In the second group, they listed the true motivators, all of them much more personal and related to the effects of the job. Their motivators include achievement, recognition, challenging work, advancement and personal growth. The existence of these motivators causes polarised feelings of satisfaction or no satisfaction – but not dissatisfaction. Although modified, the factors identified by Herzberg *et al.* are similar to those in Maslow's hierarchy:

MASLOW	HERZBERG *et al.*
Self-actualisation Esteem or status	Challenging work, achievement, personal growth, responsibility, advancement, recognition
Affiliation or acceptance Security or safety Physiological needs	Status, interpersonal relationships, supervision, policy and administration, working conditions, job security, salary

As with Maslow, Herzberg *et al.*'s research has also been challenged. The methods have been questioned, claiming that they prejudice the results (Bobbit and Behling 1972), and other researchers using different methods have found no evidence to support the two-factor theory (Locke and Whiting 1974; Ondrack 1974).

Discussion Points

Do you think that Maslow and Herzberg *et al.* reflect all the factors involved in motivation?

Make a list of the things that motivate you at work. Do they fit into Maslow and Herzberg *et al.*'s elements?

What are the differences between being dissatisfied and being demotivated?

Vroom

With Maslow and Herzberg *et al.* both appearing to be failing to describe motivation in a satisfactory way, a third theory was developed by Victor Vroom (1964). Vroom called this the expectancy theory. The basic premise of Vroom's theory is that motivation develops in proportion to the anticipated worth that an individual places on a goal and the chances he or she sees of achieving it. That is, if someone wants to achieve something that is very important to them, and they think that it may be possible, they will be highly motivated to try to achieve it. Vroom formulated his theory as:

$$\text{Force} = \text{valence} \times \text{expectancy}$$

Force refers to motivation and valence to the strength of the preference for an outcome; expectancy can be thought of as the probability that a specific action will lead to the desired outcome. If the individual does not care either way about the outcome, there is a valence of zero, and if the individual does not actually *want* to achieve the goal there is a negative valence. Both of these situations would result in no motivation. There would also be no motivation if the expectancy were negative.

Vroom's expectancy theory goes a lot further than the simple 'list of needs' approaches of Maslow and Herzberg *et al.* by recognising the importance of varying individual needs and motivations. Vroom's theory seems to reflect the complexity and unpredictability of real-life situations. However, it is precisely this recognition of the variables affecting motivation that makes Vroom's theory very difficult to apply in practice (Koontz and Weihrich 1988).

Porter and Lawler (1968) built upon expectancy theory to develop a more complete model of motivation, which goes a step further in reflecting the complex influence of motivation on working life. This model maintains that the amount of effort put into an activity depends upon the value of the reward, together with the amount of energy a person believes is required and the probability of actually getting that reward. This can be thought of as, 'Is the end product worth all this effort?' The perceived effort and the probability of actually getting the reward are also influenced by past performance in similar circumstances. This means that if people know that they can do a job, or have done it before, they have a better appreciation of the amount of effort required and the likelihood of success. If the end product is considered to be a worthwhile result, if the likelihood of reaching it is favourable and if the person has done something similar in the past with a positive result, the motivation to go ahead and make it happen will be high. Porter and Lawler's model, although complex, is probably the most adequate description of motivation. It demonstrates that motivation is not a simple cause and effect but relies upon a range of interconnecting factors.

It seems that people's actual performance is determined by effort, but their performance is also influenced by individual ability (knowledge and skills) to do the job and the perception of what the task is (understanding goals, required activities and so on). Successful performance is seen as leading to a combination of intrinsic rewards such as accomplishment and self-actualisation, and extrinsic rewards such as status and pay. These two types of reward, together with the knowledge of operating within an equitable situation, will bring satisfaction.

Motivation

Motivation is, in this model, determined by more measurable factors and also by the sense of equity – in effect, what does the individual consider to be a fair reward for the effort? And does this square with the rewards that others are getting for similar effort? The application of equity theory has a direct relationship to some leaders, particularly nurse executives. In my own research (forthcoming), and in that of Ball (1997), it is clear that many nurse executives do not consider themselves to be fairly rewarded in comparison with other executive directors, which affects their satisfaction. However, it does not always affect their motivation to stay in a job. For satisfaction to occur, there needs to be a balance between the rewards and efforts of different individuals doing similar work. Stacey-Adams (1963) has a very straightforward formula for describing this:

$$\frac{\text{outcomes by a person}}{\text{inputs by a person}} = \frac{\text{outcomes by another person}}{\text{inputs by another person}}$$

Certain inequalities may be tolerated for some time (Cosier and Dalton 1983), but prolonged feelings of inequity can result in strong reactions to a minor event.

Discussion Points

Consider the introduction of clinical grading. Was that perceived to be an equitable system?

Did the differentials introduced by clinical grading have an effect on satisfaction and motivation? Why did it have the effects it did?

Reinforcement theory also relates to motivation. Skinner (1969), discussed in Nye (1992), developed an approach to motivation called positive reinforcement. Briefly, Skinner claims that individuals can be motivated by the proper design of their workplace and by praise for their performance, and that punishment for poor performance produces negative results. Skinner's approach is to analyse the environment and the behaviour of workers and, as a result of this, to try to eliminate the identified troublesome aspects of and obstructions to performance. Workers are involved in the setting of goals and objectives, and regular feedback is given. Performance improvement is rewarded with praise. Although this seems simple, there are reports of its success in practice (Hamner and Hamner 1983). Thus positive reinforcement and giving praise has become a widespread approach to employee motivation.

Current understanding of motivation has been enhanced by McClelland's work between 1955 and 1980. He felt that there are three basic motivating needs:

1. the need for power
2. the need for affiliation
3. the need for achievement.

In simple terms, the need for power is described as a desire to influence and control, the need for affiliation as deriving pleasure from being liked and welcomed into a social group, and the need for achievement as an intense desire for success coupled with an equally intense fear of failure.

McClelland (1975) sees a high need for power as a prerequisite for the filling of leadership positions, but he concedes that ways of measuring power are crude and imprecise. He also distinguishes between self-seeking power concerns and socialised power concerns, or between power for the benefit only of the wielder and power that brings benefits for others.

In more recent studies of leadership motivation patterns (McClelland and Boyatsis 1982), consideration was given to the relative importance of need for power, the need for affiliation and the need for achievement at different levels in organisational settings. The findings demonstrated that a high need for achievement appeared to predict success for lower-level managers, and a combination of moderate to high need for power and low need for affiliation appeared to predict success at most other levels. When testing these findings in different types of organisation – technical and professional organisations as opposed to industrial environments – Cornelius and Lane (1984) found that high affiliation needs were apparent in managers considered to be good leaders.

Further work supporting McClelland's three-need theory has been carried out by Miner (1982), who studied those most frequently promoted and found a high desire for power, a high desire to compete with their peers and a positive attitude towards authority. Miner (1982) found that power motives were particularly important predictors of success. Miner and Crane (1981), studying professionals, suggest that success is predicted by a preference for professional rather than hierarchical rewards – for example, a support for education rather than an increased status. This fascinating area is certainly worth a much more detailed examination. If one believes that stability in leadership is important, longevity in particular jobs is an element that needs to be studied: if we can find out how to keep people happy and motivated in leadership positions, this can only be good news.

Motivation is a crucial issue when considering the future of leadership. My own research (Girvin, forthcoming) among nurse executives has shown that they do not necessarily fit with standard patterns. For example, above there was an indication that professionals are motivated by attention to their education and development rather than the harder elements of status and so on. My research shows quite clearly that their own development and education come almost bottom of a list of motivators for nurse executives and being able to exercise power and influence positively comes near the top. Also, their need for affiliation appears to be high as a motivating factor. At the top of the list in my research is a good relationship with the chief executive – although this may also be related to power – closely followed by a good relationship with other executive colleagues. The research is not yet published, but the findings are proving to be extremely interesting and are raising many further questions that need to be investigated.

After this brief journey through the history and development of different types of leadership theory, Chapter 8 will look at what leadership actually means in practice and the range of skills that will help us to achieve effective leadership behaviour.

References

Albarn-Metcalfe B (1989) What motivates managers? An investigation by gender and sector of employment. *Public Administration*. **67**: 95–108.

Ball J (1997) *Nurse Executives' Pay – A Survey for the Royal College of Nursing*. RCN. London.

Bobbit HR and Behling O (1972) Defence mechanisms as an alternate explanation of Herzberg's motivator-hygiene results. *Journal of Applied Psychology*. January: 24–7.

Burns JM (1978) *Leadership*. Harper & Row. New York.

Cornelius ET and Lane FB (1984) The power motive and managerial success in a professional-oriented service industry organisation. *Journal of Applied Psychology*. **69**: 32–9.

Cosier RA and Dalton DR (1983) Equity theory and time: a reformulation. *Academy of Management Review*. April: 311–19.

Hall D and Nougaim K (1968) An examination of Maslow's hierarchy in an organisational setting. *Organisational Behaviour and Human Performance*. February: 12–35.

Hamner WP and Hamner EP (1983) Behaviour modification in the bottom line. Cited in Hackman JR, Lawler E and Porter L (1983) *Perspectives on Behaviour*. Dryden Press. Illinois.

Herzberg F, Mausner B, Peterson R and Capwell D (1957) Job attitudes: a review of research and opinion. Psychological Services of Pittsburgh. Cited in Hackman JR, Lawler E and Porter L (1983) *Perspectives on Behaviour*. Dryden Press. Illinois.

Herzberg F, Mausner B and Snyderman B (1959) *The Motivation to Work*. John Wiley. London.

Kitching D (1993) Nursing leadership – myth or reality? *Journal of Nursing Management*. **1**: 253–7.

Koontz H and Weihrich H (1988) *Management*. McGraw-Hill. London.

Lawler E and Suttle JL (1972) A causal correlation test of the needs hierarchy concept. *Organisational Behaviour and Human Performance*. April: 265–87.

Locke EA and Whiting RJ (1974) Sources of satisfaction and dissatisfaction among solid waste management employees. *Journal of Applied Psychology*. April: 145–56.

McClelland D (1975) *Power: The Inner Experience*. Irvington. New York.

McClelland D and Boyatsis R (1982) Leadership motive pattern and long term success in management. *Journal of Applied Psychology*. **67**: 737–43.

Mackie L (1987) The leadership challenge. *Senior Nurse*. **6**(4): 23.

Maslow A (1954) *Motivation and Personality*. Harper & Row. London.

Miner JB (1982) The uncertain future of the leadership concept: revisions and clarifications. *Journal of Applied Behavioural Science*. **18**: 293–308

Miner JB and Crane DP (1981) Motivation to manage and the manifestation of a managerial orientation in career planning. *Academy of Management Journal*. **24**: 626–33.

Nicholson N and West M (1988) *Managerial Job Change: Men and Women in Transition.* Cambridge University Press. Cambridge.

Ondrack DA (1974) Defence mechanism and the Herzberg theory: an alternate test. *Academy of Management Journal.* March: 79–89.

Porter LW and Lawler EE (1968) *Managerial Attitudes and Performance.* Homewood. Illinois.

Savage P (1990) NHS reorganisations, leadership styles and nursing. *Senior Nurse.* **10**(4): 6–8.

Skinner B F (1969) *Contingencies of reinforcement on theoretical analysis..* Appleton-Century-Crofts. New York. Cited in Nye R (1992) *Three Psychologies.* Brooks & Cole. London.

Stacey-Adams J (1963) Towards an understanding of inequity. *Journal of Abnormal and Social Psychology.* **67**: 422–36.

Vroom V (1964) *Work and Motivation.* John Wiley. London.

Chapter 8 Leadership Today

Having considered the information in the previous chapters, it is perhaps not too difficult to see why nursing finds leadership such a tough nut to crack. In today's health care environments, the need for strong nursing leadership is greater than ever, and we simply cannot afford to remain confused and unsure about what leadership is or ambiguous about where we find it. We must be clear about the skills that we want leaders to possess, and about how we want them to operate in order to get the best results for patients and clients, the profession and our employers.

The literature we have investigated has identified a number of factors to be considered, but it is at this point that subjectivity creeps in. What follows is a personal view of how we need to address leadership in the future, one informed by the research and other literature, talked through with friends and colleagues, and, as a result, a synthesis of the things I have read and absorbed. Even if you, as the reader, do not agree with what are highlighted as the key characteristics or the major elements of successful leadership, you will still have extended your knowledge and understanding and can draw on this to develop your own leadership skills and approaches.

There have been attempts to develop categories of leader in nursing, for example, the clinical leader, the managerial leader, the educational leader, the executive leader, even the political leader; it is very satisfying to put people and things into little boxes! Leadership in nursing is much more fluid than this suggests and really defies this kind of constraining approach. What we must concentrate on is the range of skills, abilities and characteristics required and decide which ones need to come to the fore in specific situations. For example, leaders in clinical areas will need to be educational leaders and political leaders to a great extent, and managerial leaders perhaps to a smaller extent, depending upon their wider role. Executive leaders can and must be a combination of all of these. Thus it is really a question of having a portfolio of skills and then using those skills most appropriately. As a leader, one has to 'slip' between roles all the time – sometimes having a clinical focus, sometimes one more managerial, sometimes a strategic one. Being comfortable with this 'slipping' and being adept at identifying which mode to use in a given situation is what leadership is all about.

Good leaders are not one dimensional. They have a range of skills, attributes, tools and techniques at their disposal: they are multiskilled and multifaceted.

So what are these multiple skills needed by leaders? Now that we have been through a great deal of the literature, we can begin to tease out the themes that crop up over and over again. Claire Manfredi (1996) identifies seven key elements that constantly reoccur in leadership studies:

- having and achieving goals
- initiating and implementing change
- having and using influence
- having and using power
- taking responsibility for the growth of self and others
- mentoring
- having and articulating a vision.

To this, I would add an eighth factor:

- forging and sustaining relationships.

Underpinning and running through each of these elements will be the nurses' own specialist knowledge base and, of course, personality. It is suggested that effective leadership can be identified by the articulation of a clear set of core values and a clear vision of how the organisation wants to make its mark, all of these elements being the key areas of leadership. If these skills and abilities, together with sound knowledge, can be developed, nurses will be well equipped to lead in their chosen field – be it in clinical and specialist practice, as a manager, as a teacher, as an executive or in any other chosen area.

Having and Achieving Goals

The most important thing to remember about having and achieving goals is that they really need to be shared goals. If no-one wants to go the same way, you are in trouble. Thus goal-setting must be interactive and collaborative with the people you are hoping to lead. There must be shared intentions about what is needed and what you all want to do. Being able to agree and stating quite clearly what you are going to do, what you expect others to do, and within what timescale is a crucial part of being a leader. Working towards collaboratively agreed goals can give groups a sense of purpose and a sense of belonging, and reaching those goals can be a significant motivator for people (Burns 1978; Bennis 1983; Bass 1985).

Initiating and Implementing Change

When you are developing your vision and setting your goals, what you are really doing is stating clearly your intention to change things. The one constant in today's health care environments is continuous change. Change has become a bit tedious because we see so much of it and hear so much about it. Learning about change management feels a bit passé because we have all done and seen so much of it. However, one becomes blasé at one's peril. Leadership and change are inextricably linked, so one must have a good grasp of change management approaches and the skills to bring about change. Leaders frequently find themselves working in the role of change agent (Kotter 1990) and must be able to facilitate the process.

This is not a book on change management, but there are plenty of good books available and plenty of articles about the experiences of bringing about change. Knowing how to go about encouraging change is a fundamental skill in any leadership portfolio. Patience and participation are the touchstones of achieving lasting change. You will need to prepare well, have techniques at your disposal for unfreezing old attitudes; you will need to have an understanding of why people may be concerned about change or not want to work in a different way. You will need to be credible with the people you want to bring about the change and they will need to trust you. You will need to spend time with them, helping and facilitating them to work through their concerns. You will need to be prepared to review progress and change your plans if necessary, and there must be some type of evaluation mechanism to assess whether the desired changes are actually happening. You will have to encourage the refreezing of attitudes into the new ways of working and thinking. Change management is hard work, but very rewarding when all goes well. The reading list at the end of this chapter contains books and articles about change that may be helpful.

Having and Using Influence

Being able to influence others is concerned with powers of persuasion and also with the individual's credibility in the minds of those he or she is trying to influence. The notion of credibility has been discussed elsewhere. Your knowledge base will be important, as will the ability to demonstrate your knowledge to colleagues in a way that is meaningful to them and that will enhance your credibility with them. Working with integrity and in a way that builds up trust will also help your ability to influence (Kouzes and Posner 1987). If you are working in a position where you have no formal influence – perhaps in an advisory role, outside the hierarchy – then your personality, your knowledge and the way you form and develop relationships are the tools you will have to use to gain influence. Being able to marshal salient facts, having a logical argument, a calm approach to situations, patience and perseverance and an ability to keep your frustrations under control will all help. Being respectful to others will encourage them (most of them, anyway) to be respectful in their turn and, bit by bit, you will establish your credibility with staff and colleagues and be able to influence them.

Having and Using Power

We have discussed power at some length earlier in the book, concentrating on three different types of power as being the main types available to you as a leader:

- power of position
- power of knowledge
- power of authority.

There are, of course other types of power that have been identified. French and Raven (1959) identified five types – expert, referent, legitimate, coercive and reward – and Morgan (1986) described 14 different categories. Although there are people who dislike the notion of power when applied to leadership, it is an inescapable fact that any relationship will have some kind of power dynamic within it.

Whether it is position and authority power, or knowledge or personality power, it will be there as an undercurrent. Even if you do not want to use power in leadership work, every situation you enter into that involves people at a different level in the organisation or with a different role will contain an element of power. You may not give out any power signals, but you cannot control the perceptions of your colleagues. If they *think* you are powerful, it will affect the way in which they relate and react to you. It is of vital importance to be aware of the perceptions of others and to use power, whether real or perceived, as positively and constructively as possible. If you abuse your power, people will not forget it in a hurry. They will be nervous of getting involved with you again – and you cannot afford that to happen if you want to lead colleagues forward.

Mentoring

I believe that it is the responsibility of every leader actively to encourage and support the development of other potential leaders. According to Kinsey (1986), a mentor is a person who acts as a career role model, actively guiding and encouraging the career development and training of another person (or persons). In nursing, it appears that we have come relatively late to the notion of active and positive support for those who will come after us. One of the major aims of this book is to help you to understand why nursing is in the position it is, what needs to be done and how we can do what is necessary. Throughout the book, we have seen how the lack of preparation for people going into leadership positions has been a major factor in bringing nursing to its present state. Leaders must accept their responsibilities for nurturing and helping future leaders, and make sure that they have the commitment and the abilities to do so effectively. Having mentorship skills, and planning for leader succession should be part of one's vision and intentions. Being a mentor and having a mentor, whether formally or informally, is part and parcel of leadership behaviour. It can also be extremely enjoyable!

Taking Responsibility for the Growth of Self and Others

This is partly related to the above section on mentorship but goes further than mentoring future potential leaders. In any organisation, success is today dependent upon the organisation's capacity for learning and changing in order to adapt to dynamic environments. Leaders need to take account of the educational needs of their organisation and plan for meeting them, making sure that the organisation is equipped to deal competently with changes in practice, is able to take advantage of new technologies and is eager to expand the boundaries of existing ways of working. By facilitating this, leaders help to ensure that their organisation can face the future with confidence rather than dread. Additionally, leaders should be aware of their own growth and development needs and make sure that they themselves are on a continuous learning cycle. Effective leaders will recognise the importance of continuing their own development and of learning from others with relevant experience who are successful and willing to help them.

In my research with nurse executive directors, one of the most worrying trends to appear is the lack of importance that they place upon their own development and their own need for mentorship. This is an important finding and should be explored further and acted upon. One of the interviewees actually quoted a colleague who claimed that once one reached board level, one should not need further development. Comments like this either display a gross arrogance about their own performance and capability or demonstrate a lack of insight into what it takes to continue to be an effective leader. Either way, this is a problem. Leaders need to be actively engaged in their own development and in the development and education of others.

Forging and Sustaining Relationships

Leadership is wholly concerned with relationships. Early on in this book, we talked about the development of leadership theory through personal quality, behavioural style and contingency approaches leading to a greater awareness of the importance of relationships.

Rost (1994) has some particularly interesting comments on relationships and leaders. He has no time at all for the notion that leaders are great men and women doing great things. He believes that leadership is 'about ordinary human beings forming relationships to change groups, organisations, and societies according to their mutual purposes' (Rost 1994, p. 6). He completely eschews the notion of followers, seeing the two-way relationship as one of leader and collaborator – a much more active and mutual relationship than that implied by the rather more passive term of 'follower'. Rost believes that collaborators are totally engaged in the leadership process and are a crucial part of the relationship – 'Leadership is done by leaders and collaborators working together: collaborating' (Rost 1994, p. 7). These notions of collaboration and mutuality are crucially important to the idea of successful leadership laid out in this book.

Having and Articulating a Vision

I believe that having and articulating a vision is such an important part of leadership that I am going to take some time going through this in the next chapter. This seems to be a particularly daunting area for newcomers to the leadership field. One of the questions I get asked fairly often in my role as a mentor to developing leaders is, 'How do you develop a vision?' Most people have an idea of how they want things to be, but they are not sure how that becomes a vision for the future or how to progress it. It is usually just a question of talking carefully about the individual elements of visioning so people realise that it is not as complicated or mystical as they may have been led to believe.

References

Bass BM (1985) *Leadership and Performance Beyond Expectations*. New York. Free Press.

Bennis WG (1983) Transformative leadership. *Harvard University Newsletter*. In Manfredi C (1996) A descriptive study of nurse managers and leadership. *Western Journal of Nursing Research*. **18**(3): 314–29.

Burns J M (1978) Leadership. New York. Harper & Row.

French J and Raven B (1959) The bases of social power. In Cartwright D (ed.) *Studies in Social Power*. (pp. 150–67) Ann Arbor. Michigan.

Kinsey D (1986) The new nurse influentials. *Nursing Outlook*. **34**(5): 238–40.

Kotter JP (1990) What leaders really do. *Harvard Business Review*. **68**(3): 103–11.

Kouzes JM and Posner BZ (1987) *The Leadership Challenge*. Jossey-Bass. San Francisco, California.

Manfredi C (1996) A descriptive study of nurse managers and leadership. *Western Journal of Nursing Research*. **18**(3): 314–29.

Morgan G (1986) *Images of Organisation*. Sage. Beverley Hills, California.

Rost JC (1994) Leadership: a new conception. *Holistic Nursing Practice*. **9**(1): 1–8.

Further Reading

Broome A (1997) *Managing Change – Essentials of Nursing Management Series*. Macmillan. London.

Belasco J (1990) *Teaching the Elephant To Dance*. Hutchinson Business Books. London.

Hackman R, Lawler E and Porter L (1983) *Perspectives on Behaviour in Organisations*. McGraw-Hill. London.

Heron J (1989) *The Facilitator's Handbook*. Kogan Page. London.

Moss Kantor R (1983) *The Change Masters*. Routledge. London.

Chapter 9 Vision – Foresight, Insight and Dreams

In this chapter, the terms 'the organisation' and 'your organisation' will frequently appear. This is a collective term for your workplace. It does not automatically mean a large, complex unit with a great many staff but the immediate arena in which you work and operate as a leader. It might be a team of people, a ward, a community locality. It could be a group set up for a specific purpose or task, a clinical speciality, a directorate or a complete Trust. The components for developing a vision, as for leadership, are the same however large or small the working environment may be.

A separate chapter has been devoted to having and articulating a vision because it is, in my view, a fundamental aspect of being a leader. Bennis (1989) states that a guiding vision is the first basic requirement of leadership, and it cannot be emphasised enough how important it is to have an idea of how the future might look and how you want it to look. An inspiring vision should be the driving force behind all your actions, reflecting the fundamental values of the organisation and its major strategic focus. A vision must be appropriate to the organisation and be accessible to all the people in that organisation at every level. Everyone must understand what it means for them to commit themselves to this particular picture of the future. A clearly communicated and understandable vision will tell everyone what needs to be done and the activities required of them to make it happen. Your vision should be the guide that informs the organisation's decision-making, inspires its actions and provides a focus for keeping it on track. It should underpin procedures, protocols and guidelines and form the basis upon which working standards are based.

For leaders, developing and sharing a vision is really the starting point of their influence and ability to change the *status quo*. If you can share a view of the future that is simple to understand, inspirational and focused on values and aims with which everyone can identify, you have a head start as a change agent. But how do you acquire a vision? Where does it come from?

First of all, visions are not mystical experiences that suddenly convey themselves to you all neat and tidy, finished and ready to be put in to place. Developing a vision is a very commonplace activity, using skills and information that are probably already available to most people. However, I believe there to be one differentiating factor – in order to develop a vision you need to be dissatisfied with the direction you are going in at the moment. This dissatisfaction does not have to be very great – just enough to encourage tweaking at the edges of plans and objectives, enough to try to make things different. It is this search for something better that gives us the first gentle prod into thinking about how we want it to be different and then how we can actually make it different. We begin to develop our vision for the future, for our profession, for our department, for our organisation.

Step One – Information-gathering

First, your previous and current experiences must be considered. What is happening in the organisation or in your part of it? What is working, what feels like progress, what makes people happy? Is the organisation where it needs to be? Is it respected by others, held up as a model? Is it successfully meeting the needs of its clients? Is its workforce happy and motivated? Audit your standards and survey your staff, and profile your working environment in terms of skill availability and expertise. When you have gained a sense of where the organisation is, as opposed to where it needs to be, take your investigations a stage further. Talk to other people, to colleagues within and outside the organisation. Check out your conclusions with them. Do they feel the same way? Have they identified the same issues within the organisation? Find out and read about your specialist field or area. What is best practice at the moment? What are the people at the cutting edge doing? How do you measure up to that? Is that where you need to be? Is that a good direction to go in? What are the options?

Step Two – Involve Others

When your vision for the future is beginning to crystallise around all this incoming information, and you feel comfortable talking about the situation being discovered, begin to involve the people who work with and for you. Have informal discussions in which you float your ideas past them, invite them to comment and offer their ideas and views – start to build a picture of the future together. This should be a positive, constructive picture that reflects your ambitions for the service and its clients, that reflects the deep-seated values of all the staff and that excites you when talking about it together. Look for those signs of excitement in your staff, the signals in their individual behaviour telling you that you are on their wavelength, that they understand what is needed and want to be a part of the future rather than a passenger in it.

Step Three – Check It Out

Once the stage at which these ideas are consolidating has been reached and there is a reasonable degree of informal support for this view of the future, go for more formal feedback. Present the developing vision to interested groups within the organisation. Talk it through with your clinical supervisor or manager if the stage has been reached at which you feel comfortable enough to justify your thoughts without being defensive. Use the formal structures to gain access to people who can help in progressing the vision – people who will be constructively critical and encourage you to think through everything being proposed rather than letting you get carried away on a tide of preliminary excitement.

It is important not to settle upon a direction until you feel that it is right for you and your staff. Keep checking back with people to make sure they are still committed and that the vision is shaping up in a way that keeps them excited and motivated. Ask for feedback from unrelated groups, from superiors and subordinates; send the main themes to colleagues and friends in other organisations for their comments. Constantly clarify where you are going and what you are trying to achieve. It is very easy to get side-tracked into changing the world when 'visioning' is going well.

Step Four – Tweakability

Whatever else you do, stay flexible. A vision must not be carved out of stone, set up in front of everyone with deviations prohibited. Your vision must be a broad picture of the future – comprehensive but not complex, value based but not regulatory, understandable but not simplistic. The direction must be clear and unambiguous, but the plans for getting there will need scope for review and tweaking. Always listen to new voices and ideas that arise; detours will be inevitable and are often extremely enjoyable and useful. Keep the end in sight, but vary the means if necessary.

'The Trouble with Visions...'

When interviewing nurse executives for my research, one of the issues discussed was having and articulating a vision. One of them said to me, 'The trouble with visions is that you never know if you've got the right one.' Exactly so. You have to learn to trust your instincts, your own experiences, information synthesis and intuition, and then go for it. There is no right or wrong vision, and there will be doubts along the way. If you have taken the time and been sensitive enough to be in touch with people and to reflect their values, the vision will be accessible – it will mean something to others and can be progressed. The most empowering visions are developed through an interactive process. To be empowered, people must understand what is required, and to understand the situation and their part in it, they must participate (Adair 1988). Participation itself often leads to empowerment. The vision will make a difference if it has been developed collaboratively and has shared values and intentions to change.

Making it Happen

Have no illusions, it does not matter how strongly you feel about your vision, how realistic it is or how relevant – you cannot make it happen on your own. You may be a leader and have bags of charisma, but implementing a vision is not a one-person job. It is other people who will give the vision life, who will create the reality, but you, as a leader, have a major part to play in that.

Use Yourself To Set the Tone

It is not enough to simply tell other people about the vision; you must personally demonstrate the values that the vision reflects – all the time, and with integrity and belief. This must be consistent, with no temporary lapses. If you act in a way that denies or contradicts the values in the vision, you will be quickly marked as a hypocrite and the organisation will treat your vision – and you – with cynicism and dismissive attitudes; and rightly so. You must live the vision and act as an example to others. Then you can expect the same demonstrations of those values from others; when you see those values being demonstrated, remark upon it and praise people for it.

Become a Story-teller

Tell other people that the vision is working. Find stories, no matter how small or seemingly insignificant, that demonstrate the values of the vision in action. Reflect back to staff the things they have done which show that they have acted within the guidelines of the vision – they may not always recognise it for themselves. Point it out to people, frequently and with pride in their achievements. Constantly remind people what they are working towards and draw attention to activities that move them towards those aims.

Create Collaborators

If things are going well, all the people in the team will be pursuing common aims and objectives. However, this will not necessarily be enough – particularly if you are trying to promote a vision in a large organisation where you may not be as close as you would like to people at the grass-roots level. Make sure that the people in the middle of the organisation act in support of the vision. This is a little more difficult, particularly if they do not share your understanding. You may sometimes have to use position power/authority or some other sort of leverage to get die-hards to move. Try to personally involve them in the work – delegate activities to them and generate specific objectives for them that support the vision, even if it is indirect. Use key people to talk about the vision on your behalf – choose people known to be opinion leaders or ask for willing volunteers; that way you can be sure of commitment. Try to use a combination of 'telling' mechanisms, that is, mechanisms that spread the word about your vision.

What's in it for Others?

When trying to progress something that is really a long-term programme, it is important to build in some items that will provide fairly quick feedback. In the very early stages, try to have some quick 'hits' that will move towards the longer-term objectives. A focus on the short-term is expected in today's health care services – use it to take quick actions that will support the long-term approach and give an early sense of achievement to all the collaborators.

Always be on the watch for cynics and critics – be ready for them with a positive story or a recent achievement. Keep talking and living those initial values, and keep making your expectations clear. Always try to reward people for pursuing the vision. Monitor behaviour and reward the sorts of behaviour that progress towards your aims. Give direct feedback whenever possible and use whatever is at your disposal – money, promotion, public recognition, autonomy, project work – to reward positive and constructive progress. When there are opportunities to take on staff or promote people, make sure that you are involved and try to appoint people who reflect your values and respond to your vision of the future. Begin to develop a profile of the skills, abilities and behaviours that you want to have around you and the organisation. Make sure that these are communicated to everyone.

Provide training on the vision and how to promote it; never miss an opportunity to build it into any training programme. Wherever people are gathered together, for education or for meetings, try to find an opportunity to remind them of the changes they have made, the differences they have brought about and the closer they have brought the organisation to reaching the vision.

Taking Care of Yourself

All of this can be very hard work. You will be the main driving force in the early stages, and people will look to you for support and guidance, for motivation and as a role model. Although being a leader is exhilarating when things are going well, it can be very demoralising during the less successful times. Part of being an effective leader is knowing how to manage yourself so that when times are tough and you feel like giving up, you can be resilient and robust. This means having a range of coping mechanisms to help you survive the troughs and carry on up to the next peak. It is not possible to do justice to the subject of managing yourself successfully in this book, so the reader is referred to another text in the 'Essentials of Management' series – *Managing Yourself* (Tschudin with Schober 1998). It provides a very helpful insight into a number of strategies and contains many extremely useful references.

Summary

You really do have to keep at it. It is no good producing a paper statement of vision and then expecting it all just to happen. The vision must be spelt out over and over again, so that it may inspire others to produce it. The vision will be clear about the destination of the organisation and the activities to reach it. It must be focused on the strengths of the organisation, inspire people to deliver those strengths and seek clarity in everything. Effective visions really do touch the hearts and minds of others. For a vision to be effective it must:

- be clear and challenging
- help people to make sense of chaotic situations
- be stable but open to challenge and flexible to the environment
- empower the people expected to work towards it
- prepare them for the future while learning from the past
- be delivered in the everyday detail of the work rather than just in the flowery statements
- provide guidance for everyday activity and checks and balances to work within.

If you follow these guidelines, as the vision unfolds into reality, people will increase their trust in you and their willingness to collaborate. Always remember that a vision can give confidence to people, a confidence that encourages them to believe in themselves and to believe that they can deliver dreams. It can give real meaning to their work, a purpose and something to aim for, rather than just toiling through the day.

References

Adair J (1988) *Effective Leadership*. Pan. London

Bennis WG (1989) *On Becoming a Leader*. Addison Wesley. Reading, Massachusetts.

Tschudin V with Schober J (1988) *Managing Yourself – Essentials of Management Series*. Macmillan. London.

Further Reading

Mant A (1985) *Leaders We Deserve*. Martin Robertson. London

Tappen RM (1995) *Nursing Leadership and Management – Concepts and Practice*, 3rd edn. FA Davis. Philadelphia.

Rost JC (1991) *Leadership for the 21st Century*. Praeger. Westport, Conneticut.

Afterword

We are now at the end of the book. You have examined leadership and nursing, or at least my interpretation of leadership and nursing. 'Leadership' should now be something more than just a word; you should understand what it means and have a good idea of what is required to accomplish it. There are four things that your reading of this book should have made clear:

- Leaders can be anywhere in an organisation and not just at the top or in a managerial or hierarchical position
- You can learn to be a leader
- Leadership is sometimes misunderstood and often misrepresented
- The past has its part to play in nursing and should be used to inform our present and our future.

If you want to be a leader, get to it and try – but I believe that you must have certain abilities without which effective leadership is less likely. If you do not have all of them, your leadership will vary in its success. If you do have them all, or strive to obtain them, while leading may not be easy, you will be better able to enjoy creative and constructive ways of working and enhance your chances of success. YOU can be a leader if:

- you have a vision and can inspire others with that vision
- you have goals and know how to achieve them
- you know how to initiate and implement change
- you can forge and sustain good relationships
- you can influence others
- you recognise your power and use it constructively
- you take responsibility for your own growth and development

- you take responsibility for the growth and development of others
- you act as a mentor and a role model.

Use this checklist for yourself to consider the leadership approaches of others. If everyone occupying a leadership position used this list as a template, what a great place we would be working in!

Index

Index